Fasting:
The Ultimate Diet

Fasting:
The Ultimate Diet

by Allan Cott, M.D.

with Jerome Agel
and Eugene Boe

produced by Jerome Agel

Hastings House
Book Publishers
Norwalk, Connecticut

Library of Congress Cataloging Card Number 96-076812

ISBN 0-8038-9382-5

Printed in the United States of America

10 9 8 7 6 5 4 3 2

Note

This book introduces to the public the concept of fasting as a regimen that has had beneficial effects, in cases described herein, for weight-reduction and for physical and mental problems.

Nothing in this book is intended to constitute medical treatment or advice of any nature. Moreover, as every person is adaptable to fasting in a different manner and degree, it is strongly emphasized that any person desiring to fast in even the least degree should, as for any diet, first consult his or her doctor, and should remain under the doctor's close medical supervision and advice throughout the fast and the entire period of adjustment thereafter.

—Allan Cott, M.D.

Contents

Fasting:
The Ultimate Diet

1.

Why Fast?

1. To lose weight the quickest and easiest way
2. To feel better physically and mentally
3. To look and feel younger
4. To save money
5. To give the whole system a rest
6. To clean out the body
7. To lower blood pressure and cholesterol levels
8. To cut down on smoking and drinking
9. To get more out of sex
10. To let the body heal itself
11. To relieve tension
12. To end dependence on drugs
13. To sleep better
14. To digest food better
15. To regulate bowels
16. To feel euphoric
17. To sharpen the senses
18. To quicken mental processes
19. To save time
20. To boost self-esteem
21. To learn better eating habits
22. To share with the hungry
23. To gain control of oneself
24. To seek spiritual revelations
25. To observe religious rites
26. To call attention to social issues
27. To slow the aging process

2.

All About Fasting

"I have found a perfect health, a new state of existence, a feeling of purity and happiness, something unknown to humans . . ."
—Novelist Upton Sinclair, who fasted frequently.

"The ultimate diet."

That's what fasting has been called.

Understandably so.

When you fast—when you eat nothing at all—you lose weight the quickest possible way.

This fact has the support of an unassailable mathematical logic.

This fact also has empirical support.

You may lose four or five pounds on a one-day fast.

Or up to 10 pounds on a weekend fast.

Or up to 20 pounds on a week-long fast.

Extremely obese people may lose as much as 50 percent of their weight when they go on a succession of supervised fasts.

"Fasting is a valid experience," *The New England Journal of Medicine* reported. "It can benefit any otherwise healthy person whose calories now have the upper hand in his life."

The fasting diet is a reconstructive way of life.

People have been fasting almost as long as they have been eating.

Old and New Testament figures fasted. Moses and Jesus fasted for 40 days to bring on divine revelations.

2

The golden Greeks of antiquity fasted to purify their bodies and sharpen their mental processes.

In Russia, Tolstoy and his contemporaries fasted to divert the mind from materialistic concerns and to give the stomach a rest. ("... to refuse food and drink ... is more than a pleasure, it is the joy of the soul!")

British suffragettes fasted to publicize the inferior status of women.

American Indians fasted to induce visions and dreams and to placate their gods.

Colonial New Englanders fasted to save food and discipline themselves.

Fasting enjoyed great popularity in this country during the late 19th century. In those robust days people fasted simply to give themselves a "housecleaning."

Today Americans fast for all kinds of reasons—but especially to lose weight. Some of the other reasons are to:

- Feel better.
- Cope with soaring food prices.
- Cut down on smoking and drinking.
- Enjoy an "internal shower."
- Lower cholesterol and blood pressure levels.
- Acquire new—and better—eating habits.
- Attain spiritual "highs."
- Rid themselves of a junk-food past.
- Dramatize the plight of the starving.

Dr. Yuri Nikolayev, director of the fasting unit of the Moscow Psychiatric Institute, told me when I consulted with him in Moscow that fasts are *essential* for urban populations "constantly exposed to poisonous car exhausts, factory fumes, and other toxic air pollutants."

As a doctor who specializes in treating the mentally ill, I have used fasting as an effective measure in alleviating the symptoms of schizophrenia, which my distinguished colleague Dr. Humphry Osmond calls "the disease of the future." Many patients once given up for hopeless go on "miraculously"—after a period of fasting and the adoption of new dietary regimens—to live normal lives.

But for whatever reason people fast, they lose weight and feel much better.

When I lecture, I am often asked, "Is fasting safe?"

It is certainly safe for almost everybody. Each person is adaptable to fasting in a different manner and degree.

Unfortunately, we live in a culture that equates "three squares a day" with the preservation of life itself. It is mistakenly believed that to miss a single meal would be hazardous to one's health and well-being.

Actually, our body easily adapts itself to the fasting experience. It has ample resources to nourish itself for surprisingly long periods of time. The process of nutrition continues as though food were still being consumed. Fasting, notes a colleague, "hurriedly stops the intake of decomposition-toxins and gives the organism a chance to catch up with its work of excretion . . . it helps remove the toxins in the tissues . . . causes the body to consume its excess of fat . . ."

Fasting is *not* starving.

Starving begins only after the body's reserves have been exhausted.

Most people can fast safely for a month or longer. Our body gives the signal when it is time to end the fast.

It is a mistake to regard fasting as the panacea for whatever ails you. It is even a mistake to think of it as the cure for *anything*. But there is impressive documentation, such as Dr. Nikolayev's 30 years' experience with some 10,000 fasts, that fasting allows the body to mobilize its defense mechanisms against many ills. Healing is a biological process—as much a function of life as breathing.

Four hundred years before the birth of Christ, Hippocrates, "the first man of medicine," prescribed fasting as a measure to combat illnesses. "Everyone has a doctor in him," said Hippocrates. "We just have to help him in his work." ("To eat when you are sick," he also said, "is to feed your sickness.") Often taking his own "medicine," Hippocrates lived to the ripe old age of 90.

No one would dispute the wisdom of getting plenty of rest or taking an occasional vacation. Shouldn't we treat our digestive system to a rest now and then, too? Digesting food is the toughest job our body has to contend with. When we stop eating for a time, we give the system a chance to renew itself.

Hunger, amazingly, disappears during a fast. It may seem incredible that you can completely give up eating and not feel hungry, but there is a rational explanation. As long as you are eating anything at all, the palate is in a state of stimulation . . . savoring the last meal . . . anticipating the next one. When nothing is consumed, there is no "memory" of food to titillate the taste buds. Any "hunger pangs" are mild and ephemeral. Fasting is so easily tolerated because there is no sensation of feeling hungry after the second or third day. (Even the ultra-conservative *Journal of the American Medical Association* has reported this phenomenon.)

Fasting may be a healthier way to lose weight than any of the diets that restrict you to one food or to an unbalanced combination of foods. My post-fast diet— see pages 97–107—is designed to maintain weight-control.

I cannot stress this too strongly: *You should consult your doctor before beginning even a brief fast, just as you would before beginning any diet.* A long fast, even at home, must be done under the supervision and guidance of a doctor. It is best to undergo a long fast only in a medical setting. After any fast you should have a thorough medical checkup.

Too many of us live in a limbo where we feel just "so-so" or "okay." Fasting delineates the difference between feeling "just okay" and feeling abundantly alive.

I personally have never had a weight problem (I weigh about 138 pounds and I am 5′ 7″) and I always feel well. But when I fast for just a couple of days to feel really "on top of the world," I also lose four or five pounds.

Fasts are adaptable to a busy life. On a fast of a few days, there is no need to change your schedule. You can go to work. You can keep up with your social life. You should exercise, but don't jog. I recommend long brisk walks. (There's a saying among centenarians in the remote Ecuadorian village of Vilcabamba: Each of us has two "doctors"—the left leg and the right leg.)

People of all ages and from all backgrounds are now fasting: athletes, musicians, students, teachers, union leaders, clergymen, doctors, housewives, actors, construction workers, pharmacists, artists, designers, photographers, and "the working girl." We asked some of them to share their experiences with us. The following comments are excerpted from their "testimonials" (presented in chapter 15):

> "I am [now] a human dynamo."
> ". . . a new lease on life . . ."
> ". . . no more insomnia."
> ". . . I 'recycled' my body . . ."
> ". . . never lost weight so fast . . ."
> ". . . I experience a natural 'high.' "
> ". . . this bright new future."

Research for this book involved extensive travel. We visited several places around the world that provide supervised fasting. We consulted with authorities in cities as far-flung as Buenos Aires, London, and San Antonio. In Moscow Dr. Nikolayev told me that treatment through fasting is "an internal operation without a scalpel," and William L. Esser, in Lake Worth, Florida, said that one should fast whenever one wants to feel better or look better.

Gael Greene, the biting (sic) restaurant critic of *New York* magazine, wrote us: "For a congenital gourmand, it seems easier and less painful to simply stop eating altogether rather than exercise moderation. The longest I've fasted was six days. Once for three, and now and then I fast for a day."

The vigorous actress Cloris Leachman, who sparkles as she describes herself as "sort of a mobile social worker," told CBS television viewers that she hates smoking and coffee and hard booze and sugar and meat, and that one of her solutions to the problems of the body is to fast. "Fasting is simply wonderful," she said. "It can do practically anything. It is a miracle cure. It cured my asthma."

You already fast every day of your life—between dinner and break-fast.

I hope this book will encourage you to extend your fast . . . to a full day or to a few days—or even longer.

Bon fast!

3.

It's a Discipline

Most diets are fads. They all hold out the promise of a rapid and painless shortcut to losing weight. Each has its season and is soon supplanted by the next "instant" fad to get rid of those unwanted pounds.

They come and they go:
The Mayo diet.
The grapefruit diet.
The Rockefeller diet.
The clamped-jaw diet.
The brown rice diet.
The hard-boiled egg diet.
The drinking man's diet.
The staple puncture diet.
The liquid 900-calorie-a-day diet.
The HCG-500-calorie clinic diet.
The 1000-calorie cider vinegar, lecithin, kelp, and B_6 diet.
Dr. Stillman's "quick weight loss" diet.
Dr. Atkins' "diet revolution."
And on. And on.
Senator George McGovern's Select Committee on Nutrition and Human Needs turned up no less than 51 egg and grapefruit diets.

Almost all fail. They are too restrictive and too monotonous to stick to.

In contrast to diets that are fervently embraced but soon forgotten, fasting is a discipline that has stood the test of time—*at least 5000 years.*

The thousands of people who are fasting these days

8

to lose weight rapidly discover that fasting, because it is *hunger-free*, is easier and pleasanter than being on a diet. Writing in *Playboy* magazine about his fasting experience, Malcolm Braly confessed: "I was grateful to have broken a lifelong obsession with eating."

4.

When You Fast:

You Lose Weight the Quickest Way

You are inevitably going to lose weight when you fast, even though losing weight may not be your goal.

In our weight-conscious society, however, more and more people are fasting *deliberately* to lose weight.

Is it any wonder?

We have learned from actuarial tables compiled by major insurance companies around the world that desirable weight for an adult is considerably less than average weight. The difference is about 10 pounds. One tends to live longer if one is thinner.

Some 80-million of us are overweight. More than 45-million of us can be officially classified as obese. At any given time at least 20-million of us are trying desperately to do something about our weight problem.

Annually, we spend billions of dollars to get rid of the excess baggage we carry around. We don't question the price if it's for some gadget or exotic dietary aid that promises the miracle of reducing and reshaping us overnight.

We hie ourselves to "fat farms" where the hospitality may cost a thousand dollars or more a week and where, after lots of exertion and sweating, we may drop only a couple of pounds. In the elusive quest we pay a pretty penny for supervised regimens and injections and suppressants and creams and powders and dietetic foods.

There are those who seem to make a career out of dieting. But can anything be more frustrating? All too often the lost weight "makes a comeback" when the diet is through.

When you fast, you lose weight at a rate that would seem to be impossible. You lose weight far out of proportion to your caloric deficit.

To lose one pound of fat you must burn up 3500 more calories than you consume. Most of us who lead sedentary lives do not burn up anywhere near 3500 calories *a day*. Therefore, it wouldn't seem possible to lose even one pound a day by consuming not so much as a single calorie.

But when you fast, it is not unusual to lose four or five pounds the first day and up to 10 pounds in two days.

The explanation for this equational discrepancy is quite simple:

Our bodies are mostly water. A 160-pound man is composed of about 100 pounds of water. (The rest of his weight is made up of 29 pounds of protein, 25 pounds of fat, five pounds of minerals, one pound of carbohydrates, and one-quarter ounce of vitamins.) Sodium in food causes water retention. As soon as you stop eating, *large* amounts of water are eliminated from the body. The scale does not distinguish between fat and water or bloat. A pound is a pound is a pound.

Stunning weight losses during the first days—far exceeding those of even Dr. Stillman's so-called "water diet" and Dr. Atkins' "diet revolution"—are a powerful inducement to continue the fast. My co-author Jerome Agel lost nearly eight pounds on the first day of his first fast—"it was fanfastic"—and he was not particularly overweight. (He told me later that during that fast he became aware of the hordes who eat in theatres, on television and even on the street.)

Contrary to what you may have been led to believe, calories *do* count. But in fasting there is nothing to count: no calories, no grams of protein, no grams of carbohydrates. And there is nothing to weigh.

Craig Claiborne, the esteemed food and restaurant critic, wrote in *The New York Times* of his week at the

famous Montecatini Ferme in Italy where he went
"to take the waters" and lose weight. He was put on a
low-calorie diet that excluded fats, starches, all desserts
except fruit, and all alcoholic beverages. He lost six
pounds. Had he fasted, Mr. Claiborne might have lost
three times that much. (A fast also leads to a more
sensitive palate, which Mr. Claiborne would be the
first to appreciate. He might also have found it *easier*
to eat nothing at all. Low-caloric diets of 600 or 700
calories are not as tolerable as fasting: A little food
awakens hunger without satisfying it.)

"How fast can I lose weight?"

*The rate at which you lose weight is generally in
proportion to the degree you are overweight.*

Most overweight people who fast for a week can
expect to lose up to 20 pounds.

Jane Howard, the best-selling author, told me that
she lost 14 pounds in a week. Eugene Boe, a coauthor
of this book, lost 16 pounds. Bub Redhill, a New York
businessman, went from 242 to 222 pounds during his
week-long fast.

(When he fasted for six days to protest Soviet treatment of political prisoners, the nuclear physicist Andrei
Sakharov lost 17.6 pounds.)

Most overweight people who fast for two weeks can
expect to lose at least 25 pounds. A 250-pound person
can expect to lose between 30 and 40 pounds.

In a fast of four weeks or so, an overweight person
can expect to lose about 20 percent of his original
weight. A man who weighs 200 pounds on June 1, for
example, can look forward to being 160 pounds by
July 1. Harry Wills, the heavyweight boxer also known
as the Brown Panther, a contender for Jack Dempsey's
crown, would fast for one month each spring and lose
40 pounds to reach fighting trim.

Extremely obese people have lost up to 50 percent of
their weight in a series of supervised fasts. A 604-
pound Chicago man lost 70 pounds in the first 10
days; through succeeding fasts, sensibly spaced, he
lost more than 400 pounds. Another very obese man,
who wanted to be "a human being again," fasted for
14 consecutive weekends. Then he fasted one day a

week for nine months. Over the year's time he cut his weight exactly in half, going from 360 to 180 pounds.

At one time Dick Gregory weighed almost 300 pounds. He brought his weight down to 140 pounds through fasting.

British doctors are now using fasting for weight control. Dr. T. Lawlor, for example, has fasted patients for intractable obesity, at Botleys Park Hospital, Chertsey, Surrey. The patients ranged in age from 21 to 45 and were fasted up to 40 days. All of them tolerated the experience very well; a few even experienced euphoria.

At Glasgow's Ruchill Hospital researchers concluded that "total fasting is the most efficient method of reducing weight in obese patients." Dr. T. J. Thomson, a Scottish doctor who supervised the fast of a woman who lost 97 pounds through 35 weeks of fasting, observes that not only is fasting the best way to lose weight but that partial restriction of calories is ineffective.

You begin to live off your fat when fluid has been eliminated from your body. After the first heady days of the fast, the rate of weight loss naturally decreases. You slow down to a pound or two a day. But even the loss of a couple of pounds a day—following initial weight losses that are so dramatic—should be encouraging.

In the preparation of this book, my colleague Mr. Boe visited with Dr. Walter Lyon Bloom, whose pioneer work in the use of fasting to treat obesity was conducted at Piedmont Hospital in Atlanta. Dr. Bloom, now associate vice-president for academic affairs at Georgia Institute of Technology, came to fasting through his interest in fat mobilization.

In my research into obesity I found that fasting takes away the illogical idea that patients can't lose weight. My patients learned they were eating not because they were hungry. They learned they could go for a month without feeling famished. Fasting is probably the best self-disciplining practice I know. The only thing that counts in weight control is thermodynamics. It is pure, simple physics and chemistry. Weight is related primarily to balancing your energy intake with energy expenditure. Our preoccupation with eating at regular intervals has led to the misconception that fasting is not pleasurable. I have seen fasters lose as much as ten pounds in one day. What could be more gratifying, even though the loss is not fat but water.

As I said earlier, I enjoy fasting even though I am not trying to lose weight. By eating well—but in moderation—and by exercising I am able to maintain my weight and keep my waistline at 29 inches.

You may be interested to know what I eat.

For breakfast I have half a grapefruit or an orange, or the juice of either. I eat an egg twice a week and either a cooked or a granola-type cereal other mornings. I also have one butterless piece of toast with honey and a cup of decaffeinated coffee.

For lunch I have a cup of yogurt, or some nuts and figs or raisins.

For dinner I eat meat once a week and fish or fowl the other evenings. I always have a huge bowl of salad, with lots of vegetables, and usually a baked potato. In summer my dinner may consist of only a baked potato and cottage cheese and a huge Greek salad with oil and vinegar dressing. I almost never eat sweets. My dessert is a piece of cheese and an apple or a pear.

For exercise I walk a couple of miles every day, either to the office in the morning or to my home at night.

Let me stress my motto: "Less is better." And introduce a new one: "Let *them* eat cake."

President Ford asked Americans to cut down on food consumption by 5 percent. That amount is negligible, and hard to measure. But if we fasted one day a week we would be reducing our food consumption *by almost 15 percent.* Over a year's time this would add up to nearly two months of foodless days. Think of the savings in our food bills! Think how much weight we would lose!

You Feel Great

I have been blessed with good health all my life, but after a fast I am acutely aware of a sense of well-being.

My own experience is like that of so many others who observe that after even a few days of going without food they feel better physically, mentally and spiritually.

And now we are discovering what the animal kingdom has always known—fasting can be therapeutic.

Unless humans intervene, animals use nature's way to heal themselves. They find a quiet place to rest and they stop eating when they are ill. Even domesticated dogs and cats will resist strenuous efforts of worried masters to force them to eat.

So-called "dumb" cows are smart enough to quit eating when they are sick; sometimes they will keep their jaws clamped shut when cattle raisers or veterinarians try to force-feed them. Hunters have reported seeing a wounded elephant lean against a tree and watch his companions eat without joining them.

Man is the only "animal" who persists in eating when he is sick, even though he may have no appetite and food makes him nauseous. Though our ailing bodies reject food, we are still urged by everyone around us to "keep up your strength" or "build resistance"—keep eating, in other words.

The medical orthodoxy continues to take a jaundiced view of fasting, particularly as a therapeutic tool. This perplexed the late Alice Chase, who wrote on fasting for health: "The medical profession, ruling over the health of mankind, appears willing to subject the sick to the trial of all sorts of drugs, surgery, electric shock, and other forms of treatment that are experimental, even heroic—and sometimes useless. They are unwilling to open their minds and eyes to the more kindly procedures such as *rest of the body, mind and emotions*"—which fasting provides.

The orthodoxy opposes the treatment of the sick by non-medical practitioners. It has used its muscle to put many of these "healers" out of business. But under the supervision of naturopaths and hygienists many sick people have fasted and recovered from really serious ailments after their doctors had all but given up on them. Fasting and new eating habits were just what the doctor *hadn't* ordered.

But even when something appears to work, the profession is still not impressed. The "cure" has to be proved according to orthodox guidelines. Empirical data are not acceptable and scientific journals will not publish papers based on such data; the material is dismissed as "anecdotal."

To me it is even more regrettable that so many of my colleagues are not even interested in investigating something new that has been found to yield desirable results. But when the medical profession shifts gears from treating sickness to preventing sickness—and *it must!*—I have every confidence that fasting will be increasingly prescribed.

People who have chronically abused their bodies with too much food and the wrong kinds of food say that after their first fast they felt really well for the first time that they could remember.

Here again we can take a lesson from the animals. Many species—hedgehogs, bears, woodchucks, female polar bears—hibernate for months without a morsel of food. Birds and beasts of prey get along nicely without food for two weeks or longer. Dogs have fasted for 60 days. Fishes, turtles, and salamanders can go without food for even longer periods of time. But the record may be held by some species of reptiles; they can survive for a whole year without eating. (Tadpoles and caterpillars fast before they become frogs and butterflies.)

The incredibly energetic salmon takes no nourishment as it fights its way upstream to spawn. The journey may last for months and take it through 3000 miles of rapids and waterfalls.

In common with salmon, people discover they have amazing resources of energy during—*and after*—fasting. When we lose a lot of weight, we are naturally go-

ing to feel more energetic because our strength isn't being sapped carrying around all that "waste" poundage.

While fasting, Dick Gregory ran in the Boston Marathon. In England a man named Park Barner ran in the
52½-mile "double marathon," from London to Brighton, on a stomach that had been completely empty for
24 hours. "Not only did he finish without having his
energy run dry," the magazine *Runner's World* reported,
"he ran almost a half hour faster than his previous best
for 50 miles. Two weeks later, in a 36-miler, he used
the same fasting technique. He passed the marathon
mark within minutes of his best time at that distance,
and went on another ten miles at the same pace." In
the days when the University of Chicago had a football
team, Anton Carlson, the distinguished professor of
physiology, discovered that a fast of three or four days
before a game usually increased the energy and endurance of the players.

Dick Gregory has proposed a provocative idea for
the rehabilitation of prisoners, many of whom suffer
from malnutrition. "Prisoners who engage in purifying
fasts," he advocates, "could be credited with good-
behavior time. The penal system that initiates these
suggestions just might find it is on top of a tremendous
breakthrough in the area of rehabilitation. It just might
find that difficulties in rehabilitation stem more from the
jailhouse kitchen than from any other source."

Fasting is a calming experience. It is restful. It
relieves anxiety and tension. It is rarely depressing and
it is often downright exhilarating. A colleague at Mount
Sinai Hospital, in New York, tells us that fasting relaxes his muscle spasms, enabling him to reach a
plateau in yoga exercises that would otherwise have
been a long time in coming.

We have long ago discarded the myth of fat people
being jolly people. We know they didn't become fat
through just the joy of eating. Anxieties usually lead to
overeating, and it is the aftermath of overeating that
brings on fresh anxieties focused on health. Quick
weight loss from fasting can dissipate these anxieties.

I don't know just how it happens, but many fears

seem to disappear or diminish after fasting. I have heard reports of people who lost their fears of flying and crowds and darkness and heights.

One of my patients, who was a recent Harvard graduate, had been a stutterer since he was three years old; on the fifth day of my prescribed fast, his stuttering stopped—and it has not recurred.

Nearly half the population (a staggering 100-million of us) complain of sleeping problems. They sometimes or always have trouble getting to and/or staying asleep. During and after a fast many insomniacs discover they are sleeping better than they have for years. This should not be surprising. Fasting, which has been described as "nature's tranquilizer," relaxes the nervous system and eases the anxieties that account for much sleeplessness. The internal organs are at rest, and this rest is conducive to sleep. Much insomnia can be traced to the consequences of overeating or eating the wrong food: heartburn, bloating, acid indigestion. Because the body operates more efficiently during and after a fast, many people find they do not *require* as much sleep as they used to.

Fasting can be a cheap "high"—the cheapest "high." A state of ketosis, difficult to distinguish from intoxication, can be reached. "Groovy" people refer to it as "a trip," a drugless road to euphoria; they seek "good vibes" and ecstatic visions. They also find that longer fasts can bring on the desired state of susceptibility to spiritual renewal. They flush out their systems and break dope and junk-food "habits." (Their mentor, Herman Hesse's Siddhartha, fasted.)

We are the most antiseptic people on Earth—externally. Others find excessive our germ-consciousness and preoccupation with cleanliness. I wish we all were as concerned with internal cleanliness. In a fast of a week or so we can get rid of toxins that accumulate from food we eat and the very air we breathe. It is a detoxifying strategy that gives the system "a clean bill of health."

Cutting down on weight is one sure way to lower blood pressure and cholesterol levels. A brief period of fasting can bring down these levels dramatically. A

28-year-old-man, as one example, lowered his cholesterol level from 232 to 165 milligrams in the three
weeks it took him to shed 35 of his 209 pounds. Follow-
up fasts help to maintain the lowered levels.

Fasting may be effective in treating many more
varieties of sickness than orthodox medical circles are
ever likely to concede. I am dismayed by the number of my colleagues who brand all naturopaths and
chiropractors and hygienists as "charlatans." On the
other hand, I am also turned off by the extreme "nat-
uralists," who claim the expertise of orthodox medicine
is totally misguided. Both groups have something to
contribute; they could be learning from each other.

All kinds of skin disorders are said to benefit from
fasting. It isn't that fasting by itself cures acne or
eczema or psoriasis. But the abstention from eating
leads the way to a refeeding diet that can discover which
foods or combinations of foods are causing the trouble.
Skin irritations are often caused by habitual overeating,
particularly of starches and sugars, or by some specific
food or foods to which the person is sensitized. Many
clear up after a cleansing fast and a new diet.

When I was in Moscow, I learned about the use of
fasting in the treatment of venereal and dermatological
diseases in the clinic of Lumumba University. At University Hospital in Lund, Sweden, researchers saw bald
patients—both men and women—start to grow hair
again after fasts of only ten days.

Sufferers from such assorted ailments as constipation, hay fever, asthma, peptic ulcers, arthritis, and
colitis avow that their symptoms either disappeared or
were greatly alleviated after a fast. I have read in the
literature that "the value of the fast for the sufferer
with hay fever and asthma is so fully established that
we can only wonder why it is not more generally resorted to."

Interestingly, *Christian Century* magazine advised its
readers to fast out of enlightened self-interest and not
"the pieties of traditional Christianity." The objective
was not to observe Lenten sacrifices but to lose weight,
improve health, and make the body more vibrant and
beautiful. "Fast because it is good for you," the maga-

zine urged; it can be an "exercise to get the body in shape to be alive to itself. This process frees the self to be more sensitive to the Creation, to ourselves, and to our histories."

Roland Crahay, professor of psychology and sociology at Warocque-Mons Institute, in Belgium, has studied the psychology of fasting, and often quotes the credo of the famous Buchinger Clinics, in Germany and Spain:

> We must restore fasting to the place it occupied in an ancient hierarchy of values "above medicine." We must rediscover it and restore it to honor because it is a necessity. A beneficial fast of several weeks, as practiced in the earliest days of the Church, was to give strength, life, and health to the body and soul of all Christians who had the courage to practice it.

(The giant Chicago-based pharmaceutical firm Abbott Laboratories published the Buchinger credo in its house organ.)

In *The Great Escape*, "a source book of delights and pleasures for the mind and body," fasting is celebrated as "the ultimate diet . . . the only one that really works, not only for losing weight but for achieving a beautiful high and for getting a look into your cosmic consciousness. Try fasting."

You Look Younger

When you lose weight, you become younger-looking and more attractive. There is no quicker way to come by these desirable effects than through fasting.

Rejuvenation is both cosmetic and real. As the pounds come off, the streamlined reflection in the mirror lifts the spirit. You begin to feel and think younger and you move to a snappier beat.

We all know that we live in a society that reveres the cult of youth—and the desire to prolong youth. Fat is regarded as ugly because it is identified with age. An effective advertising slogan states: "You weigh ten years too much."

When I fast for only two days, lines in my face seem to go away. Many people report that, after a fast, their skin takes on a better color and texture; blotches and blemishes tend to disappear; it is almost like having acquired a fresher, *earlier* version of themselves.

"The skin becomes more youthful," said Herbert M. Shelton, who fasted tens of thousands of people. "The eyes clear up and become brighter. One looks younger. The visible rejuvenation in the skin is matched by manifest evidences of similar but invisible rejuvenescence throughout the body."

In my opinion, regular fasts are far more conducive to rejuvenation than monkey- or goat-gland transplantations, hormone injections, face lifts, massive vitamin intakes, or any of the other extreme and expensive measures used "to turn back the clock."

The exterior *and* interior ravages of aging can be postponed if we periodically give our internal organs a rest and allow the body to eliminate or "burn off" its accumulations of rubbish. A more efficient metabolism acts as a rejuvenating agent.

In India a 76-year-old political dissident, Tara Singh, undertook a much publicized fast of 48 days. Afterward, examining physicians said it was their opinion that abstention from food had "increased Singh's life span by at least ten years." When he was on the tenth day of a fast, the illustrious Mohandas K. Gandhi, then 64 years old, was found physiologically to be as healthy as a man of 40.

An article in *Health* magazine stated unequivocally that if the average person were to fast one day out of every week for a whole year "he would be no older in body at the year's end than in the beginning."

On my second visit to Moscow, Dr. Nikolayev shared with me these personal comments on fasting by a man who had been fasting off and on for 50 years:

What do you think is the most important discovery in our century? The finding of dinosaur eggs in Mongolia? The radioactive watch? Television? Atomic energy? Hydrogen bombs? In my opinion the biggest discovery of our time is the ability to make oneself younger—physically, mentally, and spiritually—through rational fasting. With the help of fasting one can forget his age and thus prevent the processes of premature aging. I am 85 years old and proud of my agility. I can easily do yoga exercises standing on my head. Few people my age are able to do such exercises. I eat twice a day and never between meals. Every week I fast for 24 hours and three or four times a year for seven to ten days at a time. I believe a man can live for 120 years or more. Man does not use his common sense when it comes to food and drink and patterns of living; and then he dies too soon, not living even half his potential age. Even animals, if no one interferes, can live very long. Man is the only exception. Wild animals know how to live by instinct, what to eat and drink. But man eats the food that is most difficult to digest and drinks poisonous drinks. And then wonders why he cannot live for 100 years. In our mind we are all craving to live longer, but in practice unfortunately we are making our lives shorter. I consider physical weakness to be an insult to an instrument as marvelous as the human body. To be strong and healthy and to enjoy it—one has to work. A man can work miracles. But remember, only you can work for your health! You cannot buy it and nobody will give it to you. I am in perfect health and feel energetic all because I learned nature's laws and follow them. Fasting is the key to health; it purifies every cell in the body. I am sure that 99 percent of the sick people suffer because of improper nourishment. People simply do not understand that they litter the body by many unnatural foods, and—because of this—poisonous substances are collected in the body. If you are interested in being in good physical and mental health and in increasing vitality, start to work for this today *with nature*, not against her.

Paul C. Bragg, of California, a "life extension specialist," has fasted at least one day every week of his adult life. At the age of 85 he described himself as "a human dynamo," and was still climbing mountains. (Nine years later he is still going strong.) Mr. Bragg discovered early that even a two-day fast "will cleanse out an accumulation of toxic debris from your circulation system and vital organs so efficiently and effortlessly that you will promptly experience a powerful sense of rejuvenation of body and mind."

You Like Yourself More

Here are typical expressions of people who—by fasting—have learned they can be the master (rather than the slave) of their cravings. They reflect the return of self-esteem.

"I have never looked and felt so well in my whole life."

"It gives me a good feeling—no, it gives me a *great* feeling—to know that I am in control of myself, to know that I am no longer controlled by my appetites."

"I feel like a human being again."

A person in control of himself thinks well of himself.

Compulsive overeaters do not believe it is possible for anybody, let alone themselves, to get along without food. To them, the discovery that fasting is as easy as apple pie comes as a revelation. Self-regard, which may have been badly deflated, gets a healthy boost.

For cosmetic reasons alone, fasting is a boon to the self-image. It is much easier to like ourself when we are trim and our eyes sparkle and our skin is free of blemishes and our tongue is clean. The effects of fasting reach to the very center of our being.

Successful exertion of willpower gives us a keen sense of character-building. When we can say NO to a gratification that we have never resisted—especially to food and drink—we learn that we didn't know our own strength.

The first time most of us fast we make the amazing discovery that going without food doesn't "hurt" at all. Successive fasts become psychologically easier, too.

I believe there is enough asceticism in most of us that occasionally we get a good feeling out of denying ourself something. It gives us the chance to test our resources, to prove we need not be victims of our desires.

When we pass the test, we are entitled to reward ourself with at least a little pat on the back.

You Save Money

Most of us are aware of the health hazards and aesthetic liabilities of being overweight.

All of us are aware of the financial penalties.

In addition to all the money we spend striving to lose weight, the medical cost of becoming ill from afflictions and ailments directly traceable to overweight is already astronomical. And the cost of being sick for *any* reason may soon be out of sight.

The most economical way to get rid of excess weight is to fast.

A brief fast undertaken at home costs nothing at all. A supervised fast away from home costs only a fraction of a trip to a "fat farm"—and ensures much greater results.

You will save considerable money, as well as control your weight, if you make fasting a part of your life pattern. If you fast just one day a week, you cut your food bill by almost 15 percent (and there are continuing weight losses, another plus).

The average weekly "market basket" for feeding a family of four is going up up and away. In New York City in February 1975 the basket cost about $66. By eating nothing one day out of seven, a family of four could save over $9 a week, nearly $500 a year.

Just skipping dinner one night a week would cut more than 5 percent off your food budget.

The American Association for the Advancement of Science has predicted food-price increases of 20 to 30 percent a *year* for the remainder of the century. Not eating one or two days a week is the best way to absorb spiraling grocery bills.

During the present oil crisis we have been asked to turn down our thermostats to a healthful 68 degrees. If we choose to eat less on a day-to-day basis—or to eat nothing on some days—we would in effect be turning down our body thermostats a few degrees. By consuming less fuel (food) we also save money—and lots of it.

You Save Time

Another reward awaits you when you fast—the precious gift of found-time.

More of the day is spent in food-related activities than most of us have ever stopped to reckon.

The time it takes to eat "three squares" is the least of it.

Additional hours are also consumed in:

- Planning menus.
- Trips to the supermarket, butcher, greengrocer, baker, liquor store, and so on.
- Preparing meals.
- Setting the table.
- The cocktail hour.
- Clearing away dishes.
- Washing dishes.
- Taking out the garbage.
- Coping with food budgets.
- Anguishing over bills.

The average homemaker spends up to six hours—one quarter of the entire day—in the securing, preparing, eating, and disposing of food.

We are always saying we'd love to do this or to do that if we only had the time. Think of all the things you could do with a windfall of time. This alone is an incentive to fast. Here is a fairly pedestrian list of things to do with found-time:

- Lie in bed all day.
- Read *War and Peace*.
- See friends.
- Visit art galleries.
- Plan a vacation with money saved by fasting.
- Sit in the backyard and watch the cumulus clouds float by.
- Hike.
- Read to the blind.

- Shop for smaller-sized clothing.
- Learn Tagalog.
- Grow day lilies.
- Call Goodwill Industries.
- Enroll in a karate class.
- Meditate.
- Write poetry.
- Prepare and send to the radio telescope in San Juan, Puerto Rico, a message for transmission to extraterrestrials.
- Balance the checkbook.
- Have fun with a pocket calculator.
- Finish a game of Monopoly.
- Knock off early from the office.
- Put color photography slides in chronological order.
- Write a book on fasting.

There are millions of other things that can be done with found-time. The possibilities are as boundless as the human imagination and fancy.

Even a "half-fast" effort leads to found-time. A book editor in New York City told us that "as the day progressed, I didn't miss the skipped breakfast and rich expense-account lunch. I got lots and lots of work done, felt more energetic (and virtuous) and really had more time than I'd thought existed. Alan Lakein was right on time: Fasting is a great time-saving time whose idea has come."

Time will tell.

You Enjoy Sex More

A question I'm often asked is, "Is sex okay during fasting?"

The answer is yes, yes—but maybe not a thousand times yes.

Dr. Alberto Cormillot, whose world-famed clinic in Buenos Aires specializes in fasting obese people, told me that many of his women patients experienced an increase in sexual desires and that they tell him they "do it better."

A man in California said on NBC that when he "got involved" in fasting "one of the biggest changes was the increase in sex drive."

Losing weight enhances physical attraction. As the pounds slip away, all kinds of energies increase. Many men and women say that fasting started them on a *vigorous* sex life. Some discovered that they are sexually desirable for the very first time in their lives.

There are reports that extended fasts are beneficial for infertility. Women who were sterile are said to have conceived and impotent men to have become virile.

Fasting seems to stimulate the power of reproduction in lower forms of life. Some animals give birth during hibernation, when they are of course fasting. The aphid is rejuvenated when it stops its gluttonous habits.

It may not be too far-fetched to speculate that abstaining from food can have a restorative effect on the sexual drives and powers of reproduction of human beings.

In any event, I have yet to hear even one adverse comment about the effects of fasting on sex.

You Smoke and Drink Less

You must give up smoking and drinking while you fast. Both habits interfere with the fasting process; besides, drinking and smoking and fasting simply do not mix!

Alcoholic beverages are high in caloric content, and the consumption of any calories goes counter to the definition of fasting, of course. To drink on an empty stomach that is going to stay empty for awhile could also make you very ill. *Very.*

Smoking pollutes the body, which is also counter to the definition of fasting.

Heavy drinkers and chain-smokers do not seem to experience the painful withdrawal symptoms common to people who try to quit "cold turkey" without the support of a fast.

The body cooperates with bans on nicotine and

alcohol and other addictive habits like drug-taking and coffee-drinking.

While fasting, you probably will not even miss cigarettes or cocktails. As the body becomes "purified," there seems to be a built-in resistance to start polluting it all over again.

A week of fasting has been known to "cure" four-pack-a-day smokers.

It is a joy to know that we can take a drink or leave it alone. One midwest college professor told me that after a week's fast she had reduced her alcoholic intake from six to two drinks a day, and even to no drinks at all on many days. A writer for *Town and Country,* Lorraine Dusky, says that her fasts led to "a drastic reduction on smoking, even though I hadn't planned to cut down."

Fasting has been described as "a salvation for the man or woman who wishes to break the shackles of the poisonous habits of alcohol and nicotine." There is a "case history" of a severely disturbed woman whose central nervous system was "a shambling wreck." Every day she smoked four packages of cigarettes and drank at least a fifth of whiskey and copious amounts of coffee and tea. She was an insomniac. She had no appetite. Her thoughts kept turning to suicide. After ten months of intermittent fasting, the woman developed into a cheerful, productive person with no yearning to return to the addictive habits that had compounded her miseries.

One former heavy drinker reported that fasting drove the "devils of my former diet from my own temple" and that his life had changed completely for the better. "About three months after my first fast," he said, "I had a sip of scotch and soda and the taste was repugnant. I then remembered how bad liquor tastes to most people the first time they try it. Folks say you have to 'cultivate a taste' for booze. Even though the body is saying 'No!', people keep trying until they get used to it."

It is possible that after an extended fast the body will not *accept* unphysiologic substances like alcoholic beverages, drugs, and cigarettes. Alcoholic consumption can even be fatal if it matches the prefasting level. (Dr. Nikolayev believes that the body *cannot* accept unphysiologic substances after a long fast.)

It is my conviction that fasting gives such a sense of well-being that it is a supreme opportunity to give up *all at once*—or at least modify—dependence on alcohol, tobacco, drugs, and pills.

You Learn New, Healthier Eating Habits

E. M. Forster, one of Britain's literary immortals, observed that food is one of the five main facts of life, "a link between the known and the forgotten." It was a marvel to him that we can go on "day after day putting an assortment of objects into a hole in our faces without becoming surprised or bored."

In the course of a year the average adult eats 120 pounds of sugar, 53 pounds of fats, 100 pounds of white flour, 14 pounds of white rice, 25 pounds of potatoes, and five pounds of ice cream.

There can be no arguing that many mouths function as litter baskets and garbage dumps.

"Offending foods" cause fatigue and depression in adults. They drive children "up the wall," causing or increasing hyperactivity and interfering with their ability to learn. The Senate Select Committee on Nutrition and Human Needs was told that if sugar were being proposed today as a new food additive, its "metabolic behavior . . . would undoubtedly lead to its being banned."

A fast of a week or longer is an education. We learn that we can survive without any food for a time and that when we do start eating again it takes much less food to satisfy us.

Even our palate "reforms." We lose our taste for the sweet and the fatty and the highly processed and the synthetic. Our taste runs more to fresh fruits, vegetables, nuts, cheese, poultry, and fish. Some people become confirmed vegetarians after a fast—the thought of eating meat again even offends their aesthetic sensibilities.

After a fast—if I may be permitted a relevant pun— our overindulged appetite goes the way of all flesh.

Fasting makes food assimilation more efficient. It may be that it takes fewer calories to sustain us afterward because of the increased permeability of cell membranes.

Only about a dozen medical schools in the United States have departments of nutrition. Yet so many of the complaints that patients bring to their doctors are attributable *directly* to diet and to overweight. What we learn about nutrition so often must come from self-education.

If the medical profession were really "tuned in" to nutrition, would the waiting rooms of doctors' offices be "sweetened" with bowls of caramels and candy corn and jawbreakers and lollipops and all-day suckers? Would the corridors and the recreation rooms of hospitals be lined with vending machines purveying chocolate bars, sugary and carbonated soft drinks, potato chips, and other junk foods containing preservatives, additives, artificial coloring—with practically no nutritional value? Would cigarettes be on sale? Apples and carrot sticks and sunflower seeds and raw nuts and raisins and toasted soybeans—*that will be the day* you find *them* there!

The cliché "we are what we eat" no longer refers only to our physical being; it refers to our mental health as well. The state of nutrition affects our behavior and our mood, and can affect our sanity. The need to relate advances in the nutritional sciences to the body of medicine will soon be realized. Until the present, neither medical education nor medical practice had kept abreast of these advances. Medical teaching and thinking adhered to the narrow focus of nutritional deficiency diseases and missed the importance of diet in the creation of an optimum molecular environment for the mind.

The best hope for long-term weight control is learning to align caloric intake with energy output. A fast is an effective control. If we lapse into weight-gaining ways again, we know we now have an agreeable way of checking ourselves. Fasting, as the *Journal of the*

American Medical Association has stated, provides "the most important attribute of all—a method of self-discipline which all obese [and I will add *all people*] need and which can be repeated with beneficial effect."

Must every social occasion be marked by eating and drinking? At a funeral we bury the dead, then hurry home for refreshments. We bring food—usually the wrong kind—to the sick abed who would be better off eating nothing, let alone cakes, cookies, and candies.

A big banquet puts us to sleep—before the speaker even has a chance to. Hospitality in many parts of the country means being invited to a heavy dinner, and two hours later being served substantial snacks.

"My God," one man who had been fasting told us, "I would never have believed it possible. But there I sat drinking water all through a 'dinner' party and I probably had a better time than anybody else there. For once I really listened to what was being said, and I wasn't talking through a haze of alcohol."

In the healthiest of all possible worlds, we would follow the wisdom of the animals and eat only when we are hungry instead of eating at fixed times of the day.

Custom and social convenience dictate the hours when we eat. If it is 7:00 A.M. or noon or 6:00 P.M., it must be time for breakfast, lunch, or dinner. Many of us automatically get "hungry" around those hours.

Responding only to our body's actual needs, we would have about the same feeding schedule as babies. We would eat as many as six "meals" a day, spaced at intervals of every three or four hours. Each would be a mini-meal.

If we allowed our children to be truly self-regulatory and self-autonomous about their bodily functions, they would grow up eating only when they were hungry, as they did in their infancy. But they soon learn they must accommodate themselves to their parents' regimen of eating.

Dr. Jean Mayer, the Harvard professor of nutrition, points out that "you can become very fat by eating just one percent more than you need every day. That extra slice of bread and butter in the morning is all it takes to add a whopping ten pounds or so in a year."

No profession is more weight-conscious than show business. To project a desirable image, actors know they must stay fashionably thin. Many of them either fast or "semi-fast." One day a week Edie Adams, as an example, gives up all food and drinks only tea. Every seventh day Van Johnson confines himself to fruit juice. Octogenarian Mae West squeezes (she would!) the juice from six oranges, three grapefruits, two lemons, and adds an equal amount of distilled water; she sips this health-bearing elixir through one day a week. (It probably explains why she still has musclemen "comin' up to see her sometime.") Lynn Redgrave, who starred as the fat friend in the funny Broadway play *My Fat Friend,* is svelte in real life—now. "I've been fat," Ms. Redgrave has said, "craving food all the time . . . and now I'm thin and believe me thin is really better. I try to postpone eating until the dinner hour." Eartha Kitt eats once a day, usually at 4 P.M. The brilliant actor Sterling ("Bodily Fluids") Hayden—*Dr. Strangelove, The Killing*—has reportedly fasted up to a month. The memory expert and erstwhile professional basketball great Ejrry Aclsu stays in shape by eating only once a day and running around a lot.

The Japanese Imperial Army soldiers who came out of the jungles of the Philippines and Guam after hiding for as long as 30 years were in better shape than their countrymen back home, many of whom had grown fat in affluence. One of the soldiers ate only minute meals the whole time he was hiding out. Examining doctors declared him to be in top physical shape.

During World War II the British, whose food supplies were stringently rationed, remained remarkably fit. When food shortages eased, there was a decline in the national health and an increasing incidence of ailments that had been almost nonexistent during the siege. The countries of northern Europe had to reduce their food consumption during the War—sugar became extinct —and a decline in heart disease was noted. In Norway wheat supplies were drastically reduced—a fact that may have contributed to the astounding decrease in the number of cases of schizophrenia reported.

From the time he was a child, Thomas A. Edison

was taught to eat "just enough." He always left the dining table a little bit hungry. When his wife followed the "less-is-better" example, she became more youthful-looking and often was mistaken for her daughter.

I would be the last to lay down any arbitrary rules about when and how much we should eat. But I will say that a fast can help you get back in touch with your *real* dietary needs . . . . to appreciating the taste of real food . . . and to knowing how much of it you want and when you want it.

To skip breakfast and even lunch—to go on a mini-fast—contributes to a desirable caloric deficit. Fasting the whole day—skipping all three regular meals—hastens that caloric deficit. Caloric deficits equal weight losses.

5.
The Mentally Ill Improve

My experience with fasting mentally ill patients began in 1970 on my first visit to the Moscow Psychiatric Institute. I went there at the invitation of Dr. Yuri Nikolayev, the director of the fasting unit, who was the first to suggest that schizophrenia may be caused by a biochemical imbalance that can be corrected through the restorative powers of fasting and revised diet.

Dr. Nikolayev himself fasted several times a year in 10-to-15-day stretches. "I usually fast for prophylactic reasons," he told me. "I have fasted several times with a scientific purpose in view, to make an experiment. I always feel excellent when I fast. It is always a happy occasion and a rest for me."

Dr. Nikolayev is fond of quoting an old German proverb: "The illness that cannot be cured by fasting cannot be cured by anything else."

Fasting *per se* is not a "cure" for anything—and I can not repeat this too often—but we know that it permits the considerable healing powers of the body—and of the mind—to assert themselves. An epochal breakthrough in the treatment of schizophrenia came when Dr. Nikolayev discovered that his patients responded to the fasting treatment after all other forms of therapy had failed. The patients had been chronically ill and felt hopeless about the future. Most of them would never have functioned again. Some would have committed suicide. Many would have deteriorated and lived out the balance of their lives in the bleak back wards of a mental hospital. *Seventy percent of those treated by fasting improved so remarkably that they were able to resume an active life.*

I was particularly impressed with one of Dr. Nikolayev's successes. At the Institute there was a nuclear scientist whose case was diagnosed as senile psychosis. His memory had lapsed to the point where he could not recall his own name. But after an extended fast his memory was completely restored and he regained full possession of his intellectual powers.

The 25-day fasting treatment for schizophrenics that I instituted at New York's Gracie Square Hospital was in accordance with procedures used in Moscow.

Many patients ask if they can keep on fasting after the prescribed period. They improve so much they want to be sure their new feeling of well-being is "for keeps."

Briefly, I should like to describe one of my most rewarding "case histories":

A Canadian who had heard about my work at the hospital directed his 19-year-old son to me. The youth had had a nervous breakdown and was terrified of people and objects. He could not think clearly or concentrate. He was not capable of study. He had dropped out of the University of Toronto. He was given to hallucinations and delusions. He retreated to his bedroom. His was a classic case of schizophrenia.

Private psychotherapy and group psychotherapy were undertaken in Toronto. Drugs were prescribed. Electric shock treatment was tried. Nothing was effective. As each form of treatment failed, his depression deepened and his withdrawal from life became complete. He slept away the days. He suffered from severe, crippling fatigue. He was written off as a hopeless case.

I started him on the fasting program, and by the fifth day phased out the heavy medication he had been taking for several years. In the beginning he did not have an easy time of it. Added to his many fears and apprehensions in general was the fear he would not survive the fast. Fortunately, he made one encouraging discovery early—his appetite disappeared. Food privation was no longer a threat.

By the tenth day of his fast my patient began to have

what he described as "happy feelings." He said they were the first happy feelings he had experienced in years.

His periods of feeling well became successively longer. His fast lasted until real hunger returned, which was four weeks. He took easily to the refeeding diet.

Four years later this once "hopeless" youth still feels well and is functioning effectively. "My mind is no longer muddled," he wrote me recently, "and I feel human again."

When Dr. Nikolayev learned that I was writing this book, he asked that I share a few of his observations with my readers:

> I have pondered the paths that the fasting therapy method should follow, and concluded there are two: prophylactic and curative.
>
> Timely measures for the prevention of a disorder must be considered very important. Fasting therapy can play a key role in this aspect. Systematic short-term fasts can raise the body's reactivity and defensive forces, and they can achieve overall improvement in the patient's condition.
>
> Because the environment is constantly polluting us, fasting is essential for the arrest of the development of various chronic disorders, for the preservation of the health of following generations, and for defense against premature aging.
>
> Short-term fasting also helps to reduce the duration of mass infectious diseases, since the body's defensive powers are activated and they can more effectively fight the disease.

I should like to stress that the schizophrenic person must fast only in a medical setting.

6.

"Our Finest Hour"

"Why can't a technology clever enough to dream up a product with no nutritional value [Co-ca-Cola] find a way to get milk to famished children in a land where the cattle have died of drought?" —THE NEW YORKER

On the day the World Food Conference convened in Rome in 1974 and on the Thursday before Thanksgiving a few weeks later, about a quarter-of-a-million people fasted in the United States to underscore the plight of the millions facing hunger and death by starvation.

For most of them it was their initial experience with fasting. It gave them the feeling that it was in their power as individuals to do something to help the hundreds of millions who are threatened with extinction by famine. Moneys saved on food were sent to organizations responsible for getting emergency supplies to the hungry. We learned that we the overfed *could* share with the underfed.

The food exists now—but getting it from the lands of plenty to the famished takes money. In the future it will take money *and* a universal sense of sharing. "Our finest hour" is how a Washington Post Service writer described the possibility. "If misery remembers America in a kindly light," Colman McCarthy wrote at Christmastime 1974, "it will not be because its politicians wanted it as Number One—we were first in the number of

37

bombs, cars, and can openers—but because we were the first nation in history to decide collectively to feed the hungry at a personal sacrifice. If we aren't remembered for that, all other glories will be forgotten."

Dr. Jean Mayer has astutely observed: "The same amount of food that is feeding 210-million Americans would feed 1.5-billion Chinese on an average Chinese diet." Nobody is hungry in China these days. Furthermore, the Chinese diet is considered to be one of the healthiest in the world. In other words, it is conceivable that we could get along in good health on about *one-seventh* of the food we are now consuming if we too could muster the knack of making less go much further.

Ours is certainly the most meat-hungry society on Earth. Beefsteak is considered as much a part of our birthright as corn-on-the-cob. As the economies of western Europe and Japan boomed after World War II, the more affluent citizens also developed a taste for prime steaks. The amount of red meat a nation consumes has become an index of its prosperity.

Meat is man's most expensive and inefficient source of protein. "World reserves of food grains are just about exhausted," *The Sciences,* the magazine of the American Academy of Sciences, declared, "and we are living on current production . . . this is a precarious situation indeed . . . the ghost of Malthus has been raised again."

We all know the grim statistics. There are about 4-billion people on Earth. By the end of the century there are expected to be 7.3-billion. Of the 2.5-billion people living in the world's less developed countries, an estimated 60 percent are malnourished and 20 percent are believed to be starving.

Food production may never be able to keep pace with the increasing number of mouths to be fed. "We have just about run out of good land," Professor George Borgstrom of Michigan State University has pointed out, "and there are tremendous limitations of what we can do in the way of irrigation."

Noting that obesity is America's number one health defect, Senator Edward M. Kennedy said that while half-a-billion children are threatened with malnutrition or starvation, America "stands in ironic contrast as a land of the overindulged and excessively fed. In many ways the well-being of the overfed is as threatened as that of the undernourished."

Do we need all the protein we are consuming? Must we get *any* of our protein from red meat?

A recommendation from U.S. governmental health authorities is that men should have 56 grams of protein in their daily diet and women should have 46. Whatever amount of protein we need, we certainly do not have to be dependent on a daily consumption of chops and steaks.

Dr. John H. Knowles, president of the Rockefeller Foundation, urged that the U.S. provide the leadership in a new ethic of austerity.

The reaction of so many people who fast as a moral gesture to the starving encourages me to believe that our eating habits will change; and any change toward austerity will be a change for the better. It's a double boon, of course—the person who fasts also benefits, and in many ways.

7.

How to Fast

Drink Only Water

Strictly speaking, you are not fasting if you consume anything except water.

Even though other beverages may be calorie-free, you are better off avoiding them.

Black coffee and tea stimulate the central nervous system at a time when you are trying to give your self a rest. (I know that some doctors, including Dr. S. Heyden, of Duke University Medical Center, who supervised the fasts of 2000 obese people, permit drinking of coffee or tea during the short fast. But as long as you're fasting for even a day, why not give the nervous system a complete rest? In 1995, Dr. Heyden noted that "fasting is—at least after two–three days—even easier than keeping a low-calorie diet."

Artificially colored, flavored, and sweetened "no-cal" drinks recall the memory of food and may arouse hunger. At the same time they "poison" the digestive system and inhibit the purifying process.

Water is a faster's best friend. It facilitates the flushing of toxins and waste materials that accumulate when fatty tissue is being "burned." It keeps the body from becoming dehydrated. It also relieves those "hunger pangs" that sometimes occur at the beginning of a fast.

Man can stay alive for an astonishingly long period of time without food, providing he has water. Cloris Leachman told me that she thinks of water as "the fountain of youth."

40

I advise that you drink at least two quarts of water every day of the fast, but there is no limit to the amount of water you may drink. (There is the extreme example of a 428-pound man who drank at least five quarts of water every day while fasting.)

"If you drink two or more quarts of water a day, will some of the fluid be retained and show up on the scale as weight-gain?"

The answer is NO.

There is no reason for concern if you do not seem to be eliminating as much water as you take in. Much of the water you drink is eliminated through tens of millions of pores in your skin, which is the most dynamic organ in the elimination network.

It is best, at any time, to drink water that is not too cold. During a fast, drink mineral water if possible. Do not drink distilled water: It is the purest water you can drink, but its mineral content is zero. Ordinary tap water contains chlorine and fluorides—at the very least—and your palate at this time may find the taste of chemical additives especially offensive.

Many fasters treat themselves to an elegant goblet for their daily "diet" of two quarts of water, and they buy a case of Perrier mineral water.

During your fast you can be the life of the party as you move gingerly with your drink in hand—the ultimate watered-down drink—a glass of beautiful water.

Exercise

Contrary to popular belief, exercise does *not* stimulate appetite. An hour of exercise a day actually *reduces* appetite.

The body burns up calories faster, as we all know, when we exercise. But what is not generally known is that the body may continue to burn them up at an accelerated pace for as long as 24 hours *afterward.*

If the object of your fast is to lose weight, you will lose it that much more quickly by adhering to a daily exercise program.

I tell everybody who fasts under my supervision that

exercise is a must. I recommend brisk daily walks—up to three hours if at all possible. (And no pressing the nose against bakery or restaurant windows.)

During a fast of two or three days there is no reason why you cannot play golf or bowl or go bicycling—if that is your normal form of exercise. But you should not do anything as strenuous as long-distance running or jogging during your fast because they are sustained activities. Yes, I know that people do run in the Marathon while fasting, but I don't recommend it.

If you have been fasting for a week or longer, you may not wish to participate in activities with sudden movements.

Ease into It

I realize that most people do not consult their doctor before starting a fast, any more than they do before starting a diet.

But why not be on the safe side? Have a checkup before you fast.

The usual practice is just to start "doing it." A person makes up his mind that he is going to fast—and that's that, period. He wakes up one morning, skips break-fast —and the fast is launched.

Some people, however, need to "psych" themselves up. They "practice" by missing a meal or two for a couple of days. Or they feel they must indulge themselves in one homeric "last supper" on the eve of the fast. I certainly don't endorse a stuffing orgy, but if it takes one to *stop* eating it may be justified. It only means you start the "trip" with even more "baggage."

Take a positive approach. If it is your first fast, set your mind to experiencing it to the fullest. The average healthy person should have no apprehensions. Your attitude should be that you are going to enjoy it, as well as benefit from it—because you will.

New York magazine's sybaritic Gael Greene, who likes fasting, notes that though one experiences nobility, moral superiority and a pleasant euphoria in a long fast, "it does take a certain kind of motivation to psych yourself into the mood to fast." My advice is, if it's your first fast and you're wary: Try a one-day fast. It's a way of getting "the hang of it." A fast on a Monday after a weekend of partying works wonders—and will demonstrate how easy it all is. It gets even easier.

Start the fast with a purgative or laxative. It gives you a feeling of being "cleaned out" right away.

It is best to turn a cool ear to the warnings and dire predictions of your friends. The salubriousness of fasting is a concept still not universally embraced, in spite of its history.

Ignore observations such as "You look pale" or "You'll get sick." These are highly subjective comments, merely reflecting the fears of the people who express them. You may be cranky on the first day, but wait until you weigh yourself the next day! Watching yourself "scale down" each morning is so exhilarating that you will wonder why you ever hesitated.

Talk to people who have already fasted. Read the "testimonials" in chapter 15. The doctor who guides your fast will also be supportive.

Enjoy Your Normal Routine

A weight-loss program created by Dr. Heyden and the Duke University Medical Center has attracted much notice. It consists of fasting for 2½ days—preferably from Friday afternoon until break-fast Monday morning—and adhering to a 700-calorie-a-day diet during the work week. (The program is called the "Workingman's Diet" because it is tailored to suit the schedule, budget, and taste of the average working person.) A variation that results in even quicker weight losses is to alternate days of fasting and the 700-calorie diet.

On my second visit to the Moscow Psychiatric Institute I looked for a staff member I had become friendly with on my first visit two years earlier, in 1970. He didn't seem to be around. I finally asked for him.

I couldn't believe my eyes when the man was pointed out to me. He had been obese at our first meeting. Now he looked like a different man entirely. He was on the

25th day of a fast. Throughout the fast he had continued his full work load, and he told me he never felt better.

There is no reason for you to alter your routine, either. Your body will tell you if you're overdoing it.

As wastes are eliminated and body tones develop, you may find that you have increased resources of energy; you certainly should feel more vigorous than you do when you eat three substantial meals a day. And there's that good old proverb to ponder: "A full stomach does not like to think."

But a word of caution again: You should be careful of sudden movements, like jumping for joy or getting quickly out of bed. Quick losses of weight reduce blood-pressure levels; with fast, jerky motions this change can produce dizziness.

Do It With Others

Fasting loves company.

But not everybody is free to go to a retreat for fasting.

Fast, if you can, with your mate, lover, and/or friend so you can share the extra time meaningfully.

Join in friendly competition to see who is doing better on the scales.

Be mutually supportive.

Swap good feelings.

Stand in front of long mirrors, gazing in wonder.

Form a community fasting club.

Build a vacation around the fast.

Get lost in the great out-of-doors.

The rest is up to you.

Two of my "fast friends" had a contest when they first fasted together. They wrote down as many book, movie, play and song titles referring to "glorious food" (as it's called in *Oliver*) as they could think of. It's really amazing how many there are. Some examples: *Breakfast of Champions, A Clockwork Orange, A*

Moveable Feast, Jaws, Duck Soup, Dinner at Eight, Breakfast at Tiffany's, Tea and Sympathy, Top Banana, Milk and Honey, "The Candyman," "You're the Cream in My Coffee," "Life Is Just a Bowl of Cherries," "Little Lamb," "On the Good Ship Lollipop," Beethoven's "Fifth," "The Ladies Who Lunch," and *Grease.*

8.

Who's Fasting

Fasting is indeed an idea whose time has come.

Articles in mass circulation periodicals report that fasting "is a very good preparation for accepting a life-long program of low-calorie diet" and that it "is of great psychological value." Even women's magazines, whose revenues come largely from food advertisers, extol the virtues of fasting. Project FAST—Fight Against Starvation Today—sponsored by World Vision International —is a national endeavor.

As we were writing the last words of this book, our local media—the New York press—reported many fasting stories . . . The National Conference of Catholic Bishops called for two days of fasting a week . . . The country-western team Seals & Crofts were said to be celebrating a 19-day religious fast . . . A woman in a much publicized court case (alienation of affections) revealed that she had fasted because "I had read that fasting makes you feel more composed." . . . Bill Walton, the former U.C.L.A. basketball giant, told a *Sports Illustrated*-interviewer that he had fasted . . . A poet working in a pilot writing program in Florida prisons said, on the second day of his second fast within two weeks, that "while we are turning down the thermostats, it would be a good idea to regulate the internal controls as well, to look within, to see what we have become." He wrote for the Op-Ed page of *The New York Times* that "a day of fasting, religiously observed once a week, would be a good place to begin." (Students at New York City's most prestigious high school, Stuyvesant, argued the poet's views in class.) . . . A Taft High School basketball player said that "I'm cutting down on eating. I go a whole day without eating and of course I never eat before a game. You gotta give the digestive system a rest." . . . Fasting was also "in the air." On an NBC television game show, "Blank Check," a contestant said that he had lost 40 pounds in 10 days—by fasting, of course . . . On "Masterpiece Theatre," a doctor prescribed a two-day fast for a sick woman in "Vienna 1900."

In increasing numbers young people have rediscovered fasting. They are fasting for at least three reasons:

1. To feel better.
2. To have "good vibes."
3. To express moral indignation.

They are now sophisticated about "empty calories" and drug addiction and food additives and alcohol. Forsaking food for a time is a way to "shape up."

Teen-aged girls are prompted to fast because they realize that chubbiness is not "in." All those cola drinks and chocolate cakes and pizzas!!! An article in *Playboy* magazine described a girl at the end of a long fast: "She just seemed to glow, she was transparently beautiful."

But may I urge that young people *never* fast, not even for a day, without their doctor's approval.

There used to be a consensus that children should not fast. But after extensive investigation, researchers at Duke University concluded that children can safely fast for one or two days a week *provided* that protein intake on all the other days *exceeds* the minimum requirement. In the post-fast diet you must be sure to get at least 60 grams of protein a day, as Dr. Heyden and his Duke colleagues discovered.

Some professional colleagues of mine—particularly Drs. Marshall Mandell, of Connecticut, and William Philpott, of Massachusetts—and I fasted children with cerebral allergies in order to isolate the offending foods causing their disturbed behavior. We also fasted adult schizophrenic and physically ill patients in order to isolate the offending foods that may be producing some of their intractable symptoms. Dr. Theron G. Randolph, of Chicago's Henrotin Hospital, reported to the twenty-third General Meeting of the Japanese Society of Allergology, in 1974, on successful fasts for physical conditions such as arthritis and ulcerative colitis.

It is not unusual for people in their 80s to fast, especially if they have been accustomed to fasting. When he was 85, Paul Bragg wrote *The Miracle of Fasting*, a book that has been an inspiration to thousands. When one fasts, Mr. Bragg wrote, one "lives in agelessness."

Herbert M. Shelton, who fasted over 40,000 people at his "school" in Texas, wrote that "fasting can bring about a virtual rebirth, a revitalization of the organism." He suggested that "if we can see in fasting a means of enabling the body to free itself, not alone of its accumulated toxic load, but also of its burden of accumulated abnormal changes in its tissues, we can use this means of rejuvenation to great advantage. Recognizing its limitations and not expecting the impossible, we may still find in the fast an avenue perhaps not to eternal youth but to a protracted youth that endures long into what we once considered old age!" William L. Esser, who directed a fasting center in Florida for several decades, fasted on a regular basis, and in his "golden years" played a dynamic game of tennis. He was a glowing testimonial to the regimen he recommended.

9.

Four Illustrious Fasters

- Upton Sinclair.
- A genteel English housewife.
- Dick Gregory.
- Mohandas K. Gandhi.

These four fasted for quite different reasons. Their experiences are inspirational.

The novelist Upton Sinclair was looking "for a diet that permits me to overwork with impunity." He found it in fasting. Fasting so enriched Sinclair's long life— he lived to be 90—that he was frequently moved to rhapsodize about it:

> The first day I was extremely hungry. I felt the hunger pains that everyone suffering from dyspepsia knows well. On the second morning I felt significantly less hunger, and then, to my surprise, I no longer felt hungry. Before fasting I had headaches every day for two to three weeks. Upon starting fasting, I had a headache on the first day. I stayed out in the fresh air and warmed my body under the sun . . . The third and fourth days were the same: . . . a feeling of clarity in my brain. . . .
>
> I started to take long walks and write. But most of all I was surprised by the clarity and activity of my brain. I read and wrote much more than I could have before the fasting period. I slept well. Every day about noon I would begin to feel weak, but a massage and cold shower would restore my strength. . . .
>
> [On the seventh day of the fast] I have been about and busy every minute of the day and until late at night. I have walked miles every day and have felt no

weakness to speak of. I shall continue the fast until I feel hungry. . . .

On the 12th day I cut my fast short by drinking a glass of orange juice . . . My sensations afterward were just as interesting . . . I felt at peace and relaxed and every nerve in my brain felt like a cat taking a nap on a warm oven. My brain was more active than before, as proved by my increased reading and writing.

I had a desire to take part in physical work. Before the fasting period I went mountain climbing and walked distances only when it was necessary. Now I work out in the gym, doing exercises that before would have literally broken my back, and I do them with pleasure. I even feel the responsibility of becoming an athlete.

Before the fast I was very frail and weak; now I am strong and healthy . . . The fast is not an ordeal, it is a rest. I sometimes wonder if it is quite fair to call it "fasting" when a man is simply living upon an internal larder of fat. Above all else, it means that you must give up self-indulgent eating.

Mrs. Graham is a London housewife who discovered fasting when she was "a bit plumpish." She now fasts three and four times each year "to put my house in order."

In May 1974 she gave BBC audiences a day-by-day account of her latest fast. On the seventh day of the fast Mrs. Graham said that she genuinely regretted the thought of breaking it—she wanted to continue it another week—but she was giving a dinner party that evening and considered it poor form to be having only water while her guests were trying to eat, drink, and be merrie.

Mrs. G. decided to break the fast right on the air. She bid her audience adieu by biting into a very snappish apple. (There will always be an England.)

Dick Gregory has fasted in protest of moral, social, and political wrongs. He has found that "increased knowledge of proper diet has accompanied my deeper understanding of my vocation—participation in the struggle of human dignity." It was his idea that "a cleansing fast [was] needed by the American peace negotiators to see the truth about the Vietnam war from a clean, pure perspective."

When he appears in nightclubs and lecture halls and on college campuses and television, Gregory tells his audiences about the joy of fasting.

> One fasts for the purpose of cleaning out the system, eliminating all toxic poisons collected in the body. Fasting is detoxification of the body. It is based upon the conviction that toxemia is the basic *cause* of disease. When we continue to push food into the body, or to shoot chemicals into the body, as it seeks to heal itself, we are forcing the body to use vital energies for purposes other than the restoration of health. The best way to help the body when the symptoms of disease appear is through fasting, relieving the body of the digestive function, or taking only juices, which provide help in the process of healing. The long fast puts the entire body through a cleansing. The faster notices a heightening of ethical and spiritual awareness. There is an improvement of sex. The body requires less and less sleep because it is not involved in the constant process of exerting energy to digest food.

Gandhi, the most celebrated faster of this century, and patron saint of the modern peace movement, made headlines throughout the world by using the fast as a tactic in his non-violent campaign against British rule. He also would fast in penance for the "moral lapses" of his followers.

The Mahatma, once a barrister in South Africa, where he first fasted, was an ascetic. Since fasting can lead to heightened awareness, he felt it necessary to remind his followers that:

> . . . concupiscence of the mind cannot be rooted out simply. There is an intimate connection between the mind and the body, and the carnal mind always lusts for delicacies and luxuries. To obviate this tendency, dietetic restrictions and fasting would appear to be necessary. The carnal mind, instead of controlling the senses, becomes their slave, and therefore the body

always needs clean non-stimulating food and periodical fasting.

Fasting can help to curb animal passion only if it
is undertaken with a view to self-restraint. Some of my
friends have actually found their animal passion and
palate stimulated as an after-effect of fasts. That is to
say, fasting is futile unless it is accompanied by an in-
cessant longing for self-restraint.

In the early 1930s Gandhi wrote about a recent fast
in which there was "indescribable peace within." Ob-
serving that he had enjoyed peace during all of his fasts,
"but never so much as in this one," he said there was:

> ... undoubtedly faith that it must lead to purification
> of self and others and that workers would know that
> true Harijan service was impossible without inward
> purity ...
>
> The fast was an uninterrupted 21-days' prayer whose
> effect I can feel now. I know now . . . there is no
> prayer without fasting . . . and that fasting relates not
> merely to the palate but to all sense organs . . . Thus,
> all fasting, if it is a spiritual act, is an intense prayer or
> a preparation for it. It is a yearning of the soul to
> merge in the divine essence.
>
> My last fast was intended to be such a preparation
> . . . How far I am in tune with the Infinite, I do not
> know. But I do know that the fast has made the
> passion for such a state intenser than ever.

(In India in the spring of 1975 protest fasts were
being used by an 80-year-old Gandhian leader and
his followers to win democratic rights.)

10.

No Reason to Be Afraid

"People don't realize that the chief obstacle to fasting is overcoming the cultural and social and psychological fears of going without food. These fears are ingrained."
> —Dr. Charles Goodrich, Mount Sinai School of Medicine, New York City, who has fasted many times. (In taped conversation with Eugene Boe.)

At any suggestion to fast, some people still react with shock and indignation. Their wildest fears are instantly activated.

"A person would have to be out of his mind to fast," they exclaim. Or "Me fast? Are you serious? I don't want to die."

Many otherwise enlightened people equate fasting with starvation—and starvation with certain death. They believe it would be unhealthy to miss a single meal. But they can rationalize overeating on the theory that it lets the body store up reserves for some hypothetical "rainy day" when there will be no food to eat. What they seem not to realize is that *the body tolerates a fast far better than it does a feast.*

(Fear-inspired overeating can become a deeply ingrained, life-long compulsion—beginning in infancy and continuing often to an early grave. Frequently, it has its origin in memories of some *real* period of food privation—deep poverty or a famine or a prison or a concentration camp. One woman claimed that her obesity had its origin in the great famine in Russia in 1919. She was only a baby then, but she was stuffed with every scrap of food her mother could scrounge.)

The person who has allayed his own apprehensions about fasting may find that he still has to contend with the apprehensions of others around him.

Upton Sinclair wrote persuasively about this aspect of fasting:

> Anyone who has not read enough on the subject [of fasting] and who doesn't trust the method should not even start it.
> If possible, it should be done in the presence of a person who has fasted already. No aunts or cousins —no worry warts—who would constantly say that the person looks like death itself and that his pulse is below 30 should be present. Do not panic. Don't be anxious. I fasted for 30 days in California. On the third day I walked 15 miles and even though I had not rested I felt perfectly fine. Upon returning home, I read about an earthquake in Messina and how the survivors tore each other apart because they were so hungry. The newspapers in a fearful voice reported that the people went without food for 72 hours. I too lived without food for 72 hours. The only difference was that these people *thought* they were starving to death.

In September 1974, victims of a monstrous hurricane rioted in Honduras only a couple of days after they had run out of food. They probably rioted out of fear rather than out of real hunger.

If for any reason you have to go without food for awhile, keep in mind that the body is geared to sustain itself for long periods. *Nutrition is a constant function; it goes on whether or not we are eating.*

A graphic account of a plane crash in the snow-covered Andes is the subject of the best-selling book *Alive* by Piers Paul Read. A group of young Uruguayan athletes were en route to Chile when their pilot became disoriented and the plane hit a mountain. The survivors had an almost instant fear of starving to death. After only a couple of days their thoughts turned to cannibalizing their dead colleagues. Shortly thereafter, the thought became the deed.

The Donner party—a caravan of Midwest farmers emigrating to California in the 1840s—became snow-bound in the Sierra Nevadas. Tension and frustration led to murder—and when food ran out, to cannibalism.

The experience of Ralph Flores and Helen Klaben, whose plane plunged into the wilds of northern British Columbia, in 1963, is in sharp contrast to these tales of cannibalism. Their "crash" diet consisted of a few biscuits and melted snow: hot, cold, and boiled. It was all they had for the entire seven weeks before rescue. When their ordeal was over, they were found to be in remarkably good condition, and both of course had lost much weight: he, 51 pounds; she, 45. (Ms. Klaben later said that she had been contemplating a diet, but a plane crash was not quite what she had had in mind.)

The writer Lorraine Dusky remembers that "when I first thought of going without food, the idea seemed impossible—but after having done it for two five-day stints I have turned into a zealot. Fasting brings a multitude of rewards."

Do not be concerned if you feel any unpleasantness at the beginning of the fast. Your body is undergoing beneficial changes. Side effects such as a slight head-ache, if they occur, are "healing" signs. They are momentary, and should be regarded as blessings in disguise. However, if at any time you find your fasting experience too unpleasant, consult your doctor; you may have to break the fast.

At the end of any fast you should feel much better than you did before you began it—and probably better than you have for a long, long time.

Please keep in mind that in fasting, as in so many other endeavors, *attitude* is vitally important. You stand to benefit most if you approach this wonderful new experience in a positive frame of mind. Put all fears behind you—they are inappropriate.

11.

Fasting Is *Not* Starving

The fact that the terms "fasting" and "starving" are frequently used interchangeably reflects widespread misunderstanding.

To repeat: Fasting is *not* starving.

Fasting is a positive, elective action that confers bountiful benefits.

Starving, in contrast, is usually an involuntary wasting away through the prolonged unavailability of food or adequate amounts of food.

The word "fast" derives from *faestan* (Old English: "to abstain"). The abstention is voluntary and undertaken for beneficial effects. It is life-enhancing.

The word "starvation" comes from the Old English *sterofan,* a derivation of the Teutonic verb *sterben,* which means "to die."

A person is fasting as long as he continues to eat nothing and experiences no *real* hunger. Starvation begins when the body has consumed its spare resources, craves food, and—for whatever reason—continues to be deprived of food.

Fasting and starving have only this *in common: Food is not being consumed.*

Again: Fasting is an act of will. Starving is an imposition of fate.

When we fast, we in effect decide we are going "to live off our self" for a time. We elect to take our nourishment from the "preserves" we have been "putting up" in good supply. Starvation occurs when "the pantry has been emptied."

Surprisingly, the confusion between fasting and starving is sometimes perpetuated by the medical profession and press. Too many doctors and science writers apparently still do not appreciate that to abstain from eating for a given time is not synonymous with starvation. But Dr. George F. Cahill, Jr., of the Harvard Medical School, has noted that "man's survival [of long abstentions from food] is predicated upon a remarkable ability to conserve the relatively limited body protein stores while utilizing fat as the primary energy-producing food." (In 1995, Dr. Cahill noted that people fear fasting out of ignorance: "One- or two-day fasting is still the best way to show someone that food intake is not mandatory.")

It takes a long fast to cross the line into starvation. The body's acutely sensitive antennae will give the signal when it is time to break the fast, before starvation can begin. That time does not usually occur until at least the 25th day. The surest sign to start eating again is the return of spontaneous appetite.

12.

How Fasting Works

Nature takes good care of the body during a fast. Biochemical changes and "capital reserves" stored in the tissue combine to do the job.

In his classic *Man, the Unknown* the geneticist and Nobel Prize-winner Dr. Alexis Carrel defined the fasting process:

> Privation of food at first brings a sensation of hunger, occasionally some nervous stimulation . . . but it also determines certain hidden phenomena which are more important. The sugar of the liver and the fat of the subcutaneous deposits are mobilized, and also the proteins of the muscles and the glands. All the organs sacrifice their own substances in order to maintain blood, heart, and brain in a normal condition. Fasting purifies and profoundly modifies our tissues.

Fasting brings a welcome physiological rest for the digestive tract and the central nervous system. It normalizes metabolism. The kidney preserves potassium and sugar in the blood—an important element that assures our feeling of well-being.

Normally, the body constantly works to digest foods, eliminate wastes, fight diseases, ward off sickness, replenish worn-out cells, and nourish the blood. When there is no food to digest, it needs only a minimum of energy to carry on the other functions.

Here is, in medical terms, what happens during an extended fast of at least 25 days, based on my experience and documented by Dr. Nikolayev and his staff of biochemists:

Stage one—the first two or three days of fasting—is characterized by an initial hunger excitation. Conditioned and unconditioned secretory and vascular reflexes are sharply accentuated. The food-conditioned reflex leucocytosis is considerably increased and the electroencephalogram shows intensified electrical activity in all leads with a prevalence of fast rhythms. Excitative processes are increased and the processes of active inhibitions are relatively weakened.

Stage two—from the second or third day and extending up to two weeks—is a time of growing acidosis. It is characterized by increasing excitability of all systems concerned with nutrition and by hypoglycemia and general psychomotor depression. The person who is fasting loses his appetite, his tongue is coated with a light film, and his breath acquires the odor of acetone. Conditioned reflexes cannot be elicited, and unconditioned reflexes are greatly diminished. The food-conditioned reflex leucocytosis is sharply reduced. The EEG demonstrates a decrease in electrical activity. In this phase inhibition prevails over excitative processes. This reduction in excitation extends to the cortex and produces a state of inhibitions similar to passive sleep caused by the blocking of stimuli. Stage two ends abruptly in an acidotic "crisis."

Stage three begins when acidosis diminishes. The tongue gradually loses its white coating and the odor of acetone disappears. Unconditioned secretory and vascular reflexes remain diminished, and conditioned reflexes, including reflex leucocytosis, are absent. By the end of stage three, however, when the tongue is completely cleared and appetite is restored, secretory and vascular reflexes increase.

Fasting serves as a powerful stimulus to subsequent well-being. Acidosis provoked by fasting and its compensation reflects a mobilization of detoxifying defense mechanisms that probably play an important role in the neutralization of toxins. As the acidosis decreases, the blood sugar level rises. The pH of the blood remains constant after acidosis decreases. Other parameters of the blood continue to remain constant. Insulin levels become normal.

The biochemical dynamics during fasting are the same for healthy people and for ill people, including mentally ill people.

Controlled fasting, far from causing any irreversible alterations in the person's blood picture, stimulates a striking intensification of regenerative, and consequently of metabolic, processes. Research into the biochemical dynamics of the fast reveals the vast changes stimulated in all the systems of the body. The fasting therapy mobilizes the proteins in the body; this reaches a peak in seven days. When the recovery period begins, the protein level is found to be lower than at the beginning of the fast.

If a drop in glucose is to occur, as it occasionally does, it will happen between the third to 12th day of the fast and return to prefast levels by the 20th to 25th day. The glucose level returns to normal during the recovery period. If a person has hypoglycemia, his glucose tolerance curve should be normal at the end of the recovery period.

The hormone serotonin increases from the seventh to 15th day, and by the end of the fast the level is lower than it was in the prefasting period.

Histamine and heparin are both formed in the tissues that surround the blood vessels. During the fast large amounts of heparin are formed, which lowers the histamine level.

Albumin levels in the blood are not greatly changed during the fast.

Catecholamines in the urine of ill people are found to be lower than in normal people. During the fast an ill person's catecholamines increase and the level rises to that of the normal person. During the recovery period catecholamines increase above prefast levels. They are later maintained at normal levels.

13.

You Will *Not* Feel Hungry

Incredible as it seems, hunger may be completely absent during even an extended fast.

It is fairly common to experience "hunger pangs" at the beginning of a fast. They are a misnomer for gastric contractions or stomach spasms; the pangs are not the sign of true hunger, but the *sensation* of hunger.

It is the psychological or ritualistic aspect of eating that makes the very thought of fasting forbidding to many. *Feeling* hungry can be such a habit that the difference between "false appetite" and true hunger becomes indistinguishable.

Such "pangs" as might occur disappear after the first day or two of the fast. But on diets most people feel *constantly* hungry. As so many people have found out, it is far easier to sacrifice food altogether than to try to stick to a diet low in calories.

Studies at the University of Pennsylvania and at Piedmont Hospital in Atlanta revealed that fat people respond enthusiastically to fasting for a very simple reason: They experience no feelings of hunger. Many of them think they are "made differently" from normal people and that their weight problem is hopeless. Some are so elated by rapid weight loss—without discomfort and without a craving for food—that they plead to be allowed to go on fasting after the control period ends.

The scientific literature has reported the greater tolerance for fasting than for restrictive diets. "Fasting may be an easier way of losing weight," *Science Digest* said, "than [are the] extremely low-calorie diets." A letter to the *British Medical Journal* stated: "Fasting therapy . . . presents positive features . . . weight loss is quick, and, therefore, encouraging to a patient . . . hunger usually causes less discomfort than a diet and, at the refeeding, patients can easily tolerate an 800-calorie regimen."

How can it be, then, that you will be free of all feelings of hunger if you eat absolutely nothing for days—or for weeks?

When you eat anything at all, your gastric juices and digestive system remain in a state of stimulation. While you are still digesting the last food you ate, your palate is already looking forward to more food. When you eat nothing at all, your body steps up its production of a compound called ketones. These ketones, which are broken-down products of fatty acids, are released into the bloodstream. As they increase in quantity, they suppress the appetite. During a fast of about a month real hunger occurs when the body starts to consume its protein. The return of *hunger*—normal, natural, or instinctive hunger—is generally interpreted as a sign that it is time to begin the refeeding diet.

If you fast for a few days or for a week, you will not be truly hungry when you voluntarily break the fast. While it is pleasant to eat again—and food never tasted so good—you will feel that you could have continued your fast without discomfort. You know that it was *choice,* and not gnawing hunger, that caused you to terminate it.

Hunger is not cumulative. If you eschew food for a day or two or for five days or for even a month, you will not be penalized afterward by an insatiable appetite that won't be appeased until all those missed meals have been eaten. You will have appetite, but no feelings of being famished. You will find yourself eating more sensibly and selectively than before your fast. You *will* want to eat less—you *will* enjoy it more. You will agree that fasting is the greatest thing since sliced bread.

14.

Who Shouldn't Fast

Just as there are people who should never go on a diet, there are those who must *never* fast.

You must not fast if you have these conditions:

• Heart diseases, especially a predisposition to thrombosis
• Tumors
• Bleeding ulcers
• Cancer
• Blood diseases
• Active pulmonary diseases
• Diabetes (juvenile)
• Gout
• Liver diseases
• Kidney diseases
• Recent myocardial infarction
• Cerebral diseases

Pregnant women have been known to fast, but under most circumstances I do not recommend it. Women who have just given birth must not fast.

Elderly people come through a fast with flying colors, but here again I would sound a note of caution. If you are in the senior-citizen category and have never fasted, you are advised to make *sure* you have the blessings of your doctor.

The very thin should not fast for more than a couple of days every few months, no matter their age. This is especially true of women, who tend to mobilize their scant supply of fat too quickly, with an effect similar to diabetic shock.

Do not fast without your doctor's approval if you are under his care for any reason.

15

What It's Like to Fast

"But what's that for—the Great Fast? Why a fast—and why a Great Fast?"

"Because, Dyomusha, if you stuff your belly full it will pull you right down to the ground. You can't go on stuffing like that, you have to have a break sometimes."

"What's a break for?" Dyomka couldn't understand. He'd never had anything else but breaks.

"Breaks are to clear your head. You feel fresher on an empty stomach, haven't you noticed?"

—Alexander Solzhenitsyn

On the following pages are first-person accounts, many contemporary, some historic, that describe the benefits and pleasures of fasting.

The accounts were contributed by people, of all ages and from diverse backgrounds, who fasted for a variety of reasons. (With the exception of the "case histories" with which I am personally acquainted, the following accounts are personal opinions and experiences without my corroboration, and must not be used as a guide to fasting.)

". . . a new lease on life . . ."

Since I've come to live in the United States, I have learned that the practice of fasting, despite its great antiquity, does not seem to have much respectability in the eyes of U.S. doctors, except for its quick weight-loss potential. Most doctors seem to view the human organism as an ailing machine in periodic need of replacement parts or chemical treatments.

I recently fasted at Buchinger Clinic, in Überlingen, Germany, to deal with a bothersome touch of arthritis, and because I needed a rest, and because it doesn't hurt anyone to lose weight now and then. After the fast, I was 12 pounds lighter, I had a new lease on life, and my blood pressure was lower. The bothersome touch of arthritis was also gone.

The idea of fasting is simple enough: Reduce the burden on the body for a period and it will start putting itself back into shape. Two weeks without food is the standard stretch, and it is—surprisingly enough—painless. When one stops eating, appetite vanishes. It was no problem to pass right by those tempting pastry shops in the nearby village and to limit myself to mineral water.

Alcohol and tobacco are forbidden during a fast. But it is surprising to see how unimportant such indulgences turn out to be and how easy they are to put aside.

Having just moved office and home, I'm ripe for another fast. I'd like to lose some more weight, and I could use another good rest. If I were like Voltaire, who treated himself to periodic fasts, I would fast at home. But I like the attention the clinic gives, and I like company.

> —Mrs. Jacqueline Nelson, senior vice-president, George Nelson Company, designers and planners. (In conversation with Jerome Agel.)

". . . excellent way to cure illnesses."

I got "hip" at age 29. I am now 73. Perhaps the four most important things I have learned during the past 44 years are:
—What to eat.
—When to eat.
—When NOT to eat.
—When to fast.

I am now a vegetarian. When I fast, to feel better or lose weight, I omit everything—all food, all juices except water. I prefer to drink spring or distilled water.

Up to age 29, and before I learned to eat properly, I was subject to colds, sore throats, stomach disturbances, and other common ailments. I learned to combat these problems by not eating and by going on a water fast. Fasting permits the digestive organs to rest while the bloodstream can concentrate on healing afflicted parts. Nature is always on our side if we only cooperate. My experience is not to eat when sick or in pain.

I fast until I feel better, usually one to four days. This regimen has been completely satisfactory for me.
—Samuel E. Sternberg, Chicago.
(In a letter to Jerome Agel.)

"I still feel like a new person."

My main reason for fasting was for health. I had discomfort because of a "faulty" gallbladder, and had some liver problems. After the first couple of days of fasting, I was no longer hungry. . . .

After the fast, I felt like a new person. The yellowish color of my skin and of my eyes had left, and there no longer was a gallbladder problem. I also lost 45 pounds on a frame that had been about 75 pounds overweight.

I am enjoying good health and watching carefully what I eat. I still feel like a new person. Fasting is a healthy and wonderful experience.
—Mrs. Ann Floyd, Libertyville, Ill. (In a letter to Jerome Agel.)

". . . music to my ears."

I'm on the road with my group a couple of weeks every month, and to tell the truth I become a junkie . . . that is, I can't stay out of those junk-food emporia. Burger

this, pizza that. Convenient foods they are—convenient
to bad health! Every time I return home I fast out those
fast foods. Sometimes it takes three days to rid my
system of the toxins. Fasting is music to my ears. No
Jazz.

—Flute player, Cambridge,
Mass. (Told to Jerome
Agel.)

". . . I 'recycled' my body . . ."

The first time I fasted I did it for political reasons. Two
hundred of us were locked up together in the District
of Columbia jail after May Day 1971. We fasted to
protest high bail and various privations. Our youngest
member, barely 18, told us how to conduct our fast
and pointed out that it would have many physical benefits. Before long, the politics of the fast got lost in the
body language of it. When I got out of jail I found that
the celebratory roast beef tasted like Corfam and that
I wanted to experiment with fasting and diets.

[When I moved to] a commune in the Santa Cruz
mountains of California . . . I "recycled" my body by
means of a balanced vegetarian diet and regular fasts
lasting from three days to a week at a time, once a
month . . . Now [my body] no longer accepts foods
that do not suit its new condition . . . my taste buds
seem to have been totally transformed. Rice and vegetables taste better than a hot fudge sundae ever did. I
eat a lot less than most Americans because my body
uses food more effectively.

Experienced fasters claim that the average consumer
utilizes only 35 percent of what he eats, whereas the
recycled human can use up to 85 percent. I now fast
mainly when I feel that I'm getting out of tune with my
body or when I am injured.

Animals, of course, routinely fast when hurt, but I
never connected that fact to my own experience until
recently. I had sustained a couple of deep bone bruises

that refused to get better over a three-week period. When I fasted, for other reasons, the injuries evaporated. I assume the body's building blocks could go to work on the injuries because they were not preoccupied with the digestive process.

—Sherman B. Chickering, teacher, political activist, San Francisco. (Reporting in *Harper's* magazine, and in letters to Jerome Agel.)

"*I even like me better . . .*"

Fasting is the flip side of my normal self.

I am overreaching, in some ways compulsive, previously given to overeating—and sometimes to smoking grass, which further stimulates the appetite.

Before I fasted, I often felt out of control with my eating. I was getting along, but on uncomfortable terms. Fasting is an affirmation of self-control. I prefer it to dieting because I prefer the feeling of not being hungry when not eating. If I eat just a little food, I'm hungry all day longgggggg. My mind has properly convinced me that it doesn't matter if I don't eat—I feel and act better. I even like me better during the fast. And you will, too! As the bathing suit season approaches, fasting takes on added motivation.

—Phil Howort, theatrical agent. (Told to Jerome Agel.)

"*. . . now I can run fast . . .*"

Three years ago I had a serious case of arthritis. Not a serious case in the chronic sense, but bad enough to hamper running. I couldn't sit down for more than half an hour without getting very stiff and I could not walk without a struggle for the first twenty paces. I went on a regime of careful eating of green and fresh vegetables and salads and two ten-day fasting periods in the course of eight weeks. And now I can run fast, as you probably saw in *The Sting*. Though age 64, I don't feel like a senior citizen.

—Robert Earl Jones, actor, New York City. (In a letter to Jerome Agel.)

"... makes one proud of oneself ..."

Having the discipline to fast creates a better feeling inside one's self, and the physical expulsion of body toxins makes the human being a stronger person. It is also true that if one fasts for more than three days, he or she will experience a "high" or lightness and lose the need for excess food or sleep. Fasting makes one proud of oneself for using his mind to control his body—something most people never use their will to control.

—Lynn Goldsmith, photographer. (In a letter to Jerome Agel.)

"Let me share a secret ..."

For almost all of my 57 years—or at least since my fat childhood, when mother loaded me up with soup bowls of cereal every morning—I have tried what I think is every conceivable diet. Yes, including the Vomiting Diet —and me a fastidious lady! Not much worked, and nothing worked for long.

Recently, I had a brainstorm, which figures, for I've been for a quarter of a century a teacher and a principal in the New York City school system and I am now married to a doctor. In a flash I "figure"d it out.

Q. What made me gain weight? A. Food—swallowing it, anyway.
Q. How might it be possible to lose a lot of weight? A. Don't eat any food.

Q. What is abstinence from food called? A. Fasting.

And fasting is what I've been doing, and I love it and it loves me. It's the only diet that works. Lots of water, lots of urination, and a busy life. Let me share a secret: I feel more alive, even sexier, when I fast.

As a "foodaholic," I tend to overeat on weekends, but fasting beginning on Mondays brings me quickly back to a preferred weight and appearance. And I'm working on cutting down on weekends. But thanks to fasting, my tongue is more sensitive to food, making eating a great pleasure. I like people telling me how well I look, how trim I look, how gregarious I am.

> —Cynthia Kamen, New York City.
> (In conversation with Jerome Agel.)

"... no more insomnia."

I went away to fast for a week and came back lighter by 14 pounds—the weight, according to my home postal scale, of three Manhattan telephone books. As soon as I got home, I rushed to my closet and preened before a full-length mirror in dresses that no longer felt as if they'd shrunk. (Before the fast, I had been inching toward outright obesity.)

Fasting taught me several things. I eat much less compulsively now, and more selectively. I have a new respect and sympathy for vegetarians.

Before the fast, I used to take meprobamates almost every night, either to fall asleep or to get back to sleep if I woke in the very early morning, as often happened. Now I don't even know where those pills are—it doesn't matter, because I have no more insomnia.

I also drink a lot less. In hedonistic New York it's quite usual to be offered, and accept, six drinks a day. Now I sometimes have none at all, and never a crashing hangover.

Fasting taught me how possible it is just to say "No thanks." I also learned, literally in my gut, that food need not be the obsessive concern our gluttonous society makes it seem. I keep meaning to fast again.

—Jane Howard, author, former *Life* magazine reporter. (In *Family Circle* magazine and in conversation with Jerome Agel.)

". . . extraordinary vibrancy and health."

My death sentence was pronounced by the doctor when I was 16 years old. A generally sickly body, heart symptoms, high blood pressure, profound anemia, and —perhaps most significant of all—a very heavy family history of early death from heart failure. All added credence to the stark prognosis made by one of Pittsburgh's most prominent physicians: "You have little chance of living beyond your early twenties."

I now wonder what was going on in his mind to make such a frightening prophecy to a 16-year-old. But he may have known something about reverse psychology, for my response was, "I'll show him, I'm going to live!" I did. I have.

I began to think about my system. I began to observe its reactions and to listen to its signals. Without benefit of guidance, I experimented with diet and with exercise. I noted carefully, when I felt sick, my diet and environmental factors, and I tried to note connections between conditions and feelings of well-being. I was on the path to self-awareness. Noting the clear relationship of our heavy Friday night Jewish East European meal with the terrible chest pains that inevitably followed, I began eating more simply, a lamb chop instead of chicken with fat lokshen soup, an orange or an apple instead of sugared cinnamon compote, a celery stalk instead of overboiled canned peas. Through my student days at the Curtis Institute of Music, my army stint, and my New York Philharmonic initiation, I began feeling better and better, even though I had reached the ill-fated "early twenties."

A fellow musician introduced me to "hygienic living" and to "fasting." I began an "eliminating" diet with occasional short fasts. For many months I ate only raw fruits and vegetables. The theory that the body quickly rebalances and heals itself, once it eliminates accumulated poisons, worked for me. My body became clean, strong, supple as I added fresh air, exercise, rest, and attention to emotional problems to the new diet. I felt marvelous.

During recent years I follow a less rigid and more varied regime, but I always "listen" to my body's needs and wants. I've added meditation to my daily exercise and to my diet. My friends, conventional or otherwise, will attest to my extraordinary vibrancy and health. I outrun, outwork, and outplay many people half my age. I love and enjoy life—and I am in my 40s.

—Joseph Eger, New York City.
(In a letter to Jerome Agel.)

"... made an important discovery ..."

As a seasoned member of the "yo-yo syndrome set," I have probably tried every diet. And I do mean *every,* good for me or not, crash to craze. It was inevitable that one day I would even try the fasting diet.

I learned through a little ad in *Prevention* magazine of Villa Vegetariana, a spa in the village of Santa Maria, just outside of Cuernavaca, in Mexico. I had been a vegetarian in my youth, following the example of my parents, who were influenced by the Shavians. I went to Villa Vegetariana with the thought that it wouldn't be much of a hardship to give vegetarianism another whirl with all those luscious and exotic Mexican fruits and vegetables to munch on.

The owner, a fruitarian by the name of David Stry, suggested that I might first try and enjoy fasting. I met a guest who was fasting and enjoying it, and I read Dr.

Shelton's book *Fasting Can Save Your Life.* I decided to fast.

My decision involved finding someone on the staff with a good strong right arm to whack off the top of a coconut. Whenever I felt a hunger pang, I was allowed to sip coconut water, through a straw. Coconut water is rich in minerals and its caloric content is negligible.

Although I had been advised not to be too active while fasting, I felt just fine and saw no reason to alter my habits. I did calisthenics. I swam in the pool. I led a yoga class. I joined in the folk dancing in the evening.

I felt no lessening of energy during the five days I fasted. I continued to engage in all the pleasant activities that, frankly, made me feel as though I were a kid back at summer camp. I had a sense of exhilaration from beginning to end. I continued to enjoy myself without any feeling of hunger or deprivation, consuming only the water from one coconut per day. I even allowed myself the restful and pleasant joy of lolling in a hammock at siesta time.

I lost eight pounds—more joy!—experienced a heightened appreciation of my surroundings and a real sense of discipline, and I made an important discovery I should like to share: *Fasting can be fun!*

> —Gail Benedict, radio commentator
> and public relations consultant.
> (In a letter to Eugene Boe.)

"I don't catch colds . . ."

I was a sick man for 20-odd years—and then, in 1960, I discovered fasting. I have enthusiastically fasted in the summer each year since then.

I used to have at least one cold a month. I don't catch colds any more. My ulcer has gone away.

My business is ladies' shoes. Until I started to fast, my business was not what I would have liked it to have been. I was angry at the world, testy with customers. I was much too fat. My soul was poisoned. Thanks to fasting, my disposition is much improved, my business is much improved, and, as I say, I feel and look much better. I owe my life to fasting.

I eat no lunches, and I do a tremendous amount of walking. For six months every year I am a very good boy—a 67-year-old very good boy now—which lasts me for my annual six-month binge.

In the summer of 1974 I fasted for nine days and lost 18 pounds; two months later I had maintained the loss.

—Irving Krutoff, Brooklyn. (In conversation with and by note to Jerome Agel.)

"... see women friends more as people ..."

I have been consciously working at personal development. With the onset of a job as an engineering consultant for transportation systems, I have tried an occasional fast. Each time I felt very together, enjoyed challenging situations, became very innovative, and generally dug life.

I feel that "I am" when I fast. Also, something of a relief, I see my women friends more as people and less as sex objects. Sex has become less compulsive and more spontaneous, conscious, and pure. It feels right, better than ever, and honest.

When my body is cleansed by a fast, I feel more in touch with myself and stronger in terms of self-assertion and willpower.

I am planning to fast for increasingly longer periods of time and hopefully under ideal conditions—outdoors in sunlight and without the demands and pressures of the working situation.

I am six feet tall and now weigh 150 pounds—and feel a hundred times as together as I did when I was a strapping 210-pounder. I believe that my life, finally, is expanding in good directions. What more could anyone ask!

—Victor Blue, New York City.
(In a letter to Jerome Agel.)

". . . got firmly back on the track of light eating."

I weighed in at nine pounds, and it's been uphill for 43 years. I even gain weight while watching the sugarland scenes in *The Nutcracker* ballet. I've tried every diet and lost thousands of pounds.

This last summer I lost 25 pounds by skipping meals and eating lightly. So many people said that I looked so lovely that I really wanted to stay thin. But along came the long Thanksgiving weekend and—well, you've never seen such a food binge. (Or I hope you haven't.) All my new clothes began pulling in the wrong places and I had to reintroduce myself to recent acquaintances.

I decided I just *had* to try "the ultimate diet."

For 48 hours I ate nothing and drank lots and lots of water. I walked a lot. I even did the family laundry and—to really test my determination—made meals for my *always* hungry family. I was so busy I hardly noticed a slight nervous headache.

Fasting worked! I quickly lost six pounds and I got back firmly on the track of light eating. By week's end I was again where I wanted to be.

Now I know I can binge from time to time and quickly get back to a preferred weight.

—Toni Z. Burns, Staten Island, N.Y. (In a letter to Jerome Agel.)

". . . I experience a natural 'high.' "

I regard fasting as more a spiritual experience than a physical experience. I started fasting to rid my body of excess weight, but I quickly realized that the fast is beneficial, very, for the mind. Fasting helps me see more keenly, achieve new thoughts, intensify my feelings, and, after a few days without eating, I experience a natural "high." Fasting inspires a sense of inner discipline and a controlling head. Insight into suffering and happiness comes during the fast. I have fasted many times, from one day to six days. I first fasted to clear my body of too much food. I wanted to feel my bones, and I wanted a slender body, not one filled with weights. I fasted after months of travel around the world, wanting to cleanse myself of all I had witnessed.

I had a memorable fast on a near-deserted New Jersey island. The beach became a beautiful place. Lying in a lotus position, I let the Sun shine on my body. I could feel myself grow lighter. I meditated. As I got "into" myself, I had the feeling I could accomplish telepathic feats.

Once craving for food goes away, the mind and the leaner body seem to stop craving things that lead to negative emotions like envy *and* jealousy *and* greed *and* overriding ambition—all those things the mental health poster says: "pride, fear, and confusion."

Fasting leads to a fine, strange edge on the world. Remember that Siddhartha's only skill was "Wait and fast."

I'm still smiling.

—Janet Fine, student, Columbia Graduate School of Journalism. (In a letter to Jerome Agel.

"I am a human dynamo."

I know the great benefits I have received from fasting, and that goes for my whole family. Every week I take a 24-hour or a 36-hour fast. This I never miss! In addition, I fast from seven to ten days four times a year. Over the many years (I am 85 years old at this writing) that I have been following this schedule, I have kept myself in a superior state of health. I am a human dynamo. I get more living out of one day than the average person gets out of five. I have an unlimited amount of energy for work and play! I never get tired . . . sleepy, yes . . . but never do I get that worn-out, exhausted feeling.

. . . A great feeling of energy flowed over my body when [the pesticide] poison passed out of my body. The whites of my eyes were as clear as new snow—my body took on a pink glow—and energy surged through my body . . . I had been fasting for 19 days—yet I drove over to Pasadena, to Mount Wilson, which is 6000 feet high, and climbed the trail with absolutely no exertion. I ran most of the way down the winding trail . . . In my personal opinion, fasting is the only way to rid the body of commercial poisons found in our fruits and vegetables.

. . . By fasting, extrasensory instinct becomes very keen. The fast sharpens the mind . . . tunes you in with the gentle voice of nature. Fasting has made my inner mind alert. I know positively that my mind works sharper and better after each fast I take.

If you can fast for three to seven days, most of your troubles of food disagreeing with you will be over . . . Flesh is dumb. It has all kinds of cravings . . . but you must be the master. You must control the entire body with the mind.

—Paul C. Bragg, N.D., Ph.D., Sc.D., "life extension specialist," author of *The Miracle of Fasting*.

". . . never lost weight so fast . . ."

Cold turkey without the turkey—a horrible thought. I became overwhelmed by the moments that food succored me. A pizza at the height of an argument with my wife, Anne, probably saved our marriage. She didn't know that those long walks to cool off were .revenge binges, a vendetta—against myself. In my case, it was the Mozzarella Weapon.

To survive a fast, I thought, would demand a house call from Charlton Heston. He would throw down another commandment: "Thou shalt not eat!" But I took the big step—or the big waddle, in my case—and went the way of all flesh, all the way to the Pawling Health Manor. It's a retreat, and I surrendered.

Throughout my first fast I kept uppermost in mind the advice of Robert Gross, who was supervising my fast: "Fifteen minutes at a time," to paraphrase the successful Alcoholics Anonymous slogan, "One day at a time." And it works.

"Don't project too far ahead," Dr. Gross also cautioned. "You can get hungry just thinking about getting hungry."

It was the homecoming that made it all pay off. "Daddy, what's happened? You're so thin!" What a thing to hear your daughter say, no matter how darling and cute she is, as one comes through the door after having been away only three days at the fat farm. I was hardly thin—I had lost ten pounds—but had I been *that* "gross"?

I've been on and off diets all my life, but I'd never lost weight so fast and so painlessly. I didn't have a hunger pang the whole time. I recommend fasting to everyone. Since that first fast, I have fasted several times. As an actor, it gives me a good feeling that I can be in control of myself and to know that the frustrations and anxieties of the actor's life, no matter how often he works, no matter how often he gets to perform, no matter how often he gets paid to do his thing, can be coped with in ways other than eating b-i-n-g-e-s.

During that first fast I found that it helped to keep busy. I took several projects along with me. Another distraction, but on my last day, alas, was an invitation to dalliance. I was attractive to someone besides dear darling fantastic Anne. What a revelation! I didn't do anything about it, but it was still nice to know. . . .

> —Jerry Stiller, of the comedy team Stiller and [Anne] Meara. (In conversation with Eugene Boe.)

"My fast is a beginning . . ."

My fasting calls for justice in this world where two-thirds of humanity live in utter poverty. I organized a student fasting protest to attract public attention to the serious problems in our world of poverty, of hunger, of oppressive economic structures—especially with regard to the estimated 6-million starving people in the drought-plagued heartland of Africa.

My fasting is a tool by which I can open the eyes of man, eyes that have been shut for so long to the shame and agony that grip the lives of too, too many people today. I wrote a poem about my experience:

My Fast and the Africans

My fast was meant to break the bonds of apathy; their starving breaks the bond of life and hastens death.

My fast brings headaches and slight dizziness; their starving brings a torment to the mortal body, a constant fire.

My fast can be broken; their starvation is unrelenting.

My fast may bring applause; their starving brings looks of horror and disgust.

My fast is self-imposed; their starving leaves them bewildered, victims of the worst cancer.

My fast smacks of pride; their starving is pregnant
with shame.
My fast is a hymn, a song; their starving is a funeral
dirge, a cry that shrieks of the grave.
My fast is a plea to men; their starving is no longer
a plea but a dying demand.
My fast is a beginning; their starving is an end.

> —Brian Koehler, student, St. John's
> University. (In a letter to Jerome
> Agel.)

"I remain free of lesions . . ."

A severe case of psoriasis, contracted when I was only
nine years old, encouraged my initial interest in fasting
and natural living. I had been given no hope for a cure,
even by eminent doctors. It was just one of those things
I'd have to learn to live with, I was told.

By the time I was into my teens I was suffering almost
intolerable social ostracism and emotional distress. I
was ready to grab at any thread of hope, however
fragile. Fasting was suggested, and I fasted for a few
days at a time. I gradually changed my diet to mostly
fruits and vegetables. Between the fasts and the revised
diet, my psoriasis came under control. I remain free
of lesions; no one would ever guess that I ever had had
a horrible disease. I have been a vegetarian (no flesh
foods whatsoever) for 30 of my 46 years. My husband
has been a vegetarian for the same amount of time,
and he is healthy and vigorous at the age of 62. Our
five children have been reared in the same discipline,
and they have grown up with frequent short fasts.

> —Joy Gross, wife of Robert Gross,
> director, Pawling Health Manor,
> Hyde Park, N.Y. (In a letter to
> Jerome Agel.)

". . . I experienced the spiritual thing."

Fasting is a fabulous experience! Everybody should do it every three or four months. Or oftener. Just to get back into their head.

I was 16 years old when I had my first fast. I fasted 11 days. I guess I fasted because I wanted spiritual knowledge . . . I wanted to be free of materialistic things and get out of my body. (My friends and I used to talk about things like this when we were kids.) About the ninth day I experienced the spiritual thing. But it was after I stopped fasting that I just automatically started to "travel" when I slept . . . visiting from plane to plane, planet to planet. It's been a decade since that first fast and I'm still traveling to astral bodies, maybe every other night. Sometimes I remember the trip, sometimes I don't.

So much happened after the fast. It opened me up. I just evolved. I harnessed knowledge that was exposed to me. It gave me a different outlook on this Universe . . . on every being walking the face of this planet. It convinced me that I would have to keep trying for something I can only call "soul development," the nearest thing to perfection on this planet. It made me wish I could be completely non-materialistic. Can you blame me for looking forward to my next fast?
—Michael Altamuro, hair stylist with Charles Alfieri, Inc., New York. (Told to Eugene Boe.)

". . . a sort of rest for the people, too."

To me, it was a vacation . . . we estimated that 10,000 people came here during the [three-week] fast . . . I think the fast was a sort of rest for the people, too. You know? Oh, I could go on for days about the things

that happened in the fast that were really great! . . .
And the people learned more about Martin Luther
King and about Gandhi in that fast than if we had sat
them down for a whole year of lectures.

—Cesar E. Chavez, president, United
Farm Workers of America AFL-
CIO. (Reported by Peter Matthies-
sen in *The New Yorker*.)

It was for the farm workers' struggle that I fasted
[three times], and it is for that struggle that we ask
your help.

—Mr. Chavez. (In a letter to Jerome Agel.)

"I never saw fat go so fast."

It has been an amazing experience: the pleasure of seeing those pounds melt away. I never saw fat go so fast.

My heart was very full when I left the school and all it
has meant to thousands of guests who, like myself, went
there sick and unhappy and left with a feeling of regeneration and happiness. I do not have the tremors
anymore. If I keep on improving as I am doing, I'll soon
be back to the days of my youth. In fact, I have had a
few compliments from strangers who said, "You look
very pretty this morning," and were amazed that I was
almost 71.

The brain becomes wonderfully clear; the body grows
into a recognition of its own power; languor, disinclina-
tion to mental and physical work disappear, and one
enters upon his daily duties with a vim and energy and
a delight that betoken the possession of the perfect and
abounding health that is every man's birthright.
—Three guests, Shelton's Health School, San Antonio, Texas.

"... this new bright future."

... I came to you a large 200 pounds, with a blood sugar of 385. I had spent years as a diabetic and also as an obese person, which made my personality and my home life very, very sad. With your help I have lost 80 pounds and my blood sugar is a normal count of 120. I have God and you to thank for giving me the strength to take five fasts. What a beautiful feeling it is to have this new bright future. Everyone has been sweet and kind to me. Being at your ranch has inspired me. It has been a wonderful "Garden of Paradise" and a great Family of Togetherness. This has made me continue to have faith and strength to stay here . . . My eyes are filled with tears; time is getting closer to be leaving soon to face a new and happy world. But the tears I shed today are tears of happiness because I have had the opportunity to come down here and be under your guidance and loving care. I am now able "to look straight ahead," and not back at the past years of those horrible days and nights. I [am] sitting on a great big beautiful cloud, on top of a rainbow.

> —Guest, on eve of leaving, Esser's
> Hygienic Rest Ranch. (In note
> [shortened] to William L. Esser.)

"... self-confident for the first time ..."

This is the first time during a life-long battle with overeating that I have been able to lose weight without the aid of diet pills. Amphetamines have caused me serious side effects for many years. I had taken all sorts of treatments and seen countless doctors. I was even hospitalized last year. Nothing helped. Each time I regained more than I lost. Now I feel healthier than I can ever remember. I found energy I never knew I was capable of. I feel self-confident for the first time in my life, and I know I will never regain that weight. I arrived at the [Buenos Aires] clinic in a size 28½ pants suit. I have already shed practically 100 pounds and hope in two or three months to be wearing a glorious size 12!

—Chronic dieter. (Reported in *Town and Country*.)

". . . ladies' best beautifier . . ."

As director of a fasting center for many years, I have supervised the fasts of thousands of people, including Dick Gregory.

I fast periodically myself. There is hardly an individual alive who could not benefit from a professionally designed fast, for fasting has no peer as to the benefits it affords to physical, mental and spiritual health.

Fasting is the ladies' best beautifier—it brings grace, charm, poise; it normalizes female functions and re-shapes the body contour. During a fast, the emotional, mental, and spiritual outlook experiences a glorious upsurge and becomes re-directed!

I am often asked, "Does fasting enhance male potency?" In many cases it has accomplished just that. Sexuality is not confined, solely, to the genital organs—the body functions as a whole. No matter how exquisitely spiritual and tender our feelings are, physical disabilities—such as glandular exhaustion, fatigue and lack of energy—can well alter the course. Fasting—with colon therapy and proper diet—can correct the problems and turn back the clock.

In addition to the cosmetical, psychological, and emotional advantages of a more "tuned" body—which fasting inspires—there is the exhilaration enjoyed by even those who do not have a weight problem. There is also the "weighty" problem that is created when job and income are threatened due to the basic requirements of certain occupations. Airline stewardesses, models, actors, actresses and policemen, for example, have jobs that require regimented weight control.

When one goes into a fast, the body adjusts to new habits, correcting problems that cause constipation, high blood pressure, impotency, and the like. Men and women who reach 40 and over can be rejuvenated, and have more sex appeal.

I am often askéd, "If fasting is so good, why isn't everyone doing it?"

My response: "That's just it—fasting is so simple and inexpensive no one believes it."

Controlled fasting is one of the safest, surest ways of losing weight, regaining health, and shedding a multiplicity of aches and pains, ills, and problems that stem from faulty eating habits of an over-indulgent nation. Fasting is the *perfect* way to natural perfection.

> —Alvenia M. Fulton, health consultant, Fultonia Health Food and Fasting Center, Chicago. (In a letter to Jerome Agel.)

". . . felt peppier . . . slept more soundly . . ."

The most impressive finding [in my five-day fast, for weight reduction of course] was lack of fatigue and freedom from hunger after 48 hours. I actually felt sharper mentally, and was able to perform heavy surgical operations with skill and mental alertness equal to what I had when eating. A feeling of euphoria is noted by some people on a fast, and this was my experience. I actually felt peppier and more alert mentally. I slept more soundly than when eating regularly.

For spiritual uplift, try a fast. You will find that it draws you closer to God in prayer. It makes your character stronger by the self-discipline and humble experience of denying yourself food. The double benefit is your feeling of well-being, with a clearer eye, sharper brain, springier step, and greater efficiency for your work. It has often been said, "The man eager for success has the lean, hungry look." A bit of starvation can give you that eagerness in a hurry. Try a fast for spiritual and physical fitness.

—J. DeWitt Fox, M.D., L.M.C.C., editor, *Life and Health,* "the national health journal."

". . . rejuvenation of the stomach . . ."

. . . felt as if . . . had had a month's vacation in the mountains. The mind was unusually clear and a greater amount of mental and physical work was accomplished without fatigue . . . increased the vigor of the gastric hunger contractions to that of a young man of 20 to 25. The improvement or rejuvenation of the stomach is not a matter of subjective opinion, but a matter of objective record . . .

—Professor Anton Carlson. (As reported by *Scientific American,* 1915.)

(Professor Carlson's five-day fast was reported by Maud DeWitt Pearl in the article "Hunger Strikes an Aid to Good Health." Ms. Pearl's conclusion: "The experiment settled any doubt as to the beneficial aspects of fasting . . . Professor Carlson [well known at the time for work on the digestive system] had slept in his laboratory [at Chicago University] to facilitate record keeping; he continued to teach . . . In the case of adult healthy persons, not only would they experience a general feeling of rejuvenescence but possibly the length of life might also be increased.")

"Life . . . could be enjoyed, not just endured."

I became obsessed with the thought of food. I found that if I gave in to my fantasies to a certain extent, they actually helped me to feel more comfortable. Whenever I passed a restaurant, and there must be a million of them in New York when you are fasting, I would dream over the menu as though it were the gate to paradise. In my fantasies I gorged on pastrami sandwiches, ice cream, pizza, roast beef, chicken dinners, etc. Yet, at the same time, I felt that if I were actually face to face with a pastrami sandwich, I would not be able to eat it, and this was a very curious experience . . . After not eating for 22 days I had orange juice. It tasted like ambrosia. In fact, for quite some time after the fast I found my taste buds were very sensitive and food tasted so much better than ever before. Although it naturally took awhile to regain my physical strength, emotionally I felt better than I can remember ever feeling. Life really seemed like something that could be enjoyed, not just endured. The best part of it for me was the wonderful feeling of freedom. With schizophrenia I felt upset and depressed most of the time without even really knowing why. I felt driven by my emotions. My mind, instead of being able to judge the reality and validity of my emotional reaction, was just being driven by my feelings. Many times I wished I were dead . . . Now, even though I have some tangled emotions to deal with, my depressions are never as deep or as long; they are a response to real difficulties. Most of the time I feel well and able to work through the problems that come up. I cannot really express how good it feels.

—Schizophrenic patient, who had been ill for 20 of her 41 years. (In a letter to Dr. Allan Cott after a fast.)

"My perspective is changing . . ."

. . . perhaps my major complaint of my illness was the feeling that my brain was not working right, not functioning spontaneously, that it was not, in fact, producing any thoughts at all. The only experience of thought I would have at such times would be my morbid brooding on my lack of thought. The clinical term for this is, I believe, poverty of ideation. This condition, I am much relieved to report, has apparently left me entirely, a fact I can attribute directly to my undergoing the fast.

There has also been an improvement in what might be termed socially related symptoms. My experiencing feelings of worthlessness when in contact with others has almost entirely subsided. I am much better at remembering and following conversations. Prefast, I would often become confused and be unable to engage intelligently in conversation.

Other complaints have also dissipated. My perspective is changing from that of a selfish child (shallow) to something much more mature and wise (deep). I am rarely depressed anymore. I believe myself to be still reaping the harvest of the fast. I liken it to a freight train gradually gaining momentum.

I experienced an incredible and wondrous sense of new birth. I became aware of myself as being a great quantity of human, emotional, raw material, which I can only liken to being re-made or reborn. I think this is a common feeling among fasters.

During the fast, my temperature and blood pressure were sub-average. Since the fast, I have been able to tolerate niacin at the rate of 2–3 grams per day with scarcely a hitch! Knock on wood. This may prove to be one of the most beneficial aspects of the fast. In the interests of life, I must do everything possible to improve my situation in all respects—organic, spiritual, psychological. As that great man Humphry Osmond would say, "No more mollycoddling."
>   —Schizophrenic who fasted for 26 days.
>   (Reporting to Dr. Allan Cott on a
>   therapeutic fast.)

"... I feel that I have a bright future ..."

When I began to drink juice during the recovery period, the world changed. Colors became brighter and thinking became easier . . . I feel that I have a bright future . . . I want to live a normal, healthy life, and I will decide later whether I shall return to school.

—27-year-old student from Poznan, Poland. (Interviewed in Moscow by Dr. Allan Cott.)

"I felt joy . . ."

I felt full of apathy. I was not concentrating, and when reading I had to read a line over and over. When I spoke to people, I could not remember what *I* had said. I felt a complete weakness in my muscles. When in the army I was punished by being isolated, I refused to eat for three days—and found that I felt better. I decided to fast or eat very little . . . the fast was terminated on the 27th day . . . my appetite gradually returned, and my spirits improved. I felt joy for the first time in a long while.

—Twenty-two-year-old schizo-phrenic patient. (Reported to Dr. Allan Cott at Moscow Psychiatric Institute.)

"The result was remarkable . . ."

During the time when I was a student in the medical institute, I suffered from chronic nephritis and none of the known European methods gave me any relief. Being disillusioned in modern medicine, I decided to go to a "school of fasting" and undergo fasting, in the city of Fukuoka, where I was born. My parents were categorically against it, but I went and fasted for eight days. The result was remarkable: the albuminuria and hematuria (from which I had suffered for many years) disappeared completely. The unpleasant feelings, of which I was so afraid before treatment, were much less than I expected. The next year my father, who was suffering chronic nephritis and hypertension, went to a school of fasting. Each of us fasted for ten days. As a result of treatment, I was cured completely: My father also noticed improvement. After being discharged from the institution, my father fasted every two to three months at home. His blood pressure lowered to almost normal. Albuminuria disappeared. From that time on my father was in good health and led an active life. I got acquainted with many other patients and kept in touch with them after treatment. Eighty percent of them told me in their letters about positive results, which convinced me once again about the effectiveness of this method. I began to advise everyone who suffered from chronic diseases to undergo the fasting treatment. I have cured with fasting patients with chronic diseases who had had no relief from drugs or injections.

> —Dr. Imamura Motoo, Japan. (Quoted by Dr. Yuri Nikolayev, Moscow Psychiatric Institute.)

"... lost 16 pounds in a week."

Before checking in at the Pawling Health Manor, in Hyde Park, New York, I tucked into a sumptuous last supper in the historic and picturesque Beekman Arms in nearby Rhinebeck and into a sumptuous buffet luncheon the next day at the same table. And then it was on to Pawling and "cold turkey" for the next seven days. I took to fasting like—well, like a duck to water.

I took long walks every day, usually to the neighboring village of Staatsburg. I became friendly with a librarian who had a "chocolate problem." I knew I had caught the hang of fasting when I could go to the general store and buy her a family-sized Hershey almond bar and not be tempted to take one wee nibble of it.

This was during a January thaw. Every day several of us gathered in a lean-to to take the mid-day winter Sun. But some of the conversation was not always conducive to keeping one's mind off food:

—"Where are you going to have your first meal when you get sprung from here?"

—"What's the name of that marvelous French restaurant on East 52nd?"

—"I can't wait to try that recipe for quick lasagna that I saw in *The News* this morning."

—"Did you hear that Shelley Winters got kicked out of here when she was caught sneaking in a pizza?"

I breezed through those waterlogged days feeling strong and chipper all the way. The most exhilarating moment of every day was the morning weigh-in. As a veteran dieter, hoping for a miracle from each year's new diet, I had never seen results like this. Or felt better. On my final trip to the scale that week I found I had lost 16 pounds.

I have now fasted four times, and I look forward to taking the fifth.

             —Eugene Boe, a coauthor of this book.

". . . can see poetry everywhere."

I first fasted on Yom Kippur, a traditional day of fasting, three years before my bar mitzvah. It was an ego trip to fast like the grownups. I fasted once a year for a few years, and then I went to pot—literally.

For about the next 15 years I led the opposite of a fasting kind of life. I finally weighed 260 pounds. I was a creature of consuming, not constricting.

I was sailing in the Greek Islands, with friends who had been to India and who meditated a lot and didn't eat often and often didn't eat at all. We talked about how Gandhi and Dick Gregory used the methodology of constriction for strength. That's how I came to fasting . . . to find a controlling device . . . to calm me down.

I fasted in France. by a little river in a valley. I was surrounded by seven mountains. I had such an organic sense of life—Sun, river, mountains. I started to think of the people I loved, and I composed love letters to them.

Fasting is resisting the simplest of temptation. It is a tool that adds an appreciation of all things that are human and natural. A faster can see poetry everywhere. (The *Village Voice* reported that a cop on the vice squad who says he fasts one day a week protects prostitutes from being assaulted by pimps.) When life goes against me, I go to the eternally beautiful things. I fast and watch the Earth revolve in and out of sight of the Sun. Oh, Bucky, where are you?

Fasting teaches appreciation. And values. And respect. We are lucky. We have a choice.
—Max (Schwartz), poet, San Francisco. (In conversation with Eugene Boe and Jerome Agel.)

Fasting
by Max (Schwartz)

Stuffing, stuffing, always they stuff, they stuff.
They grow fat stomachs.
They grow bayonets.
They grow rocket ships to the Moon.
But do they grow a simple caress?
Fasting.
What is the word fasting?
Fasting in truth is slowing
Slowing down of time
Putting time into one act of now
Putting time not into the out-there of random stupidity
Putting time into the appreciative cutting of the carrot,
The cutting of the celery, the cutting of the onion,
The serving of the tray, the giving of the glance,
The giving of the glass, the giving of the caress,
The simple time-felt being at one with the moment,
The simple time-felt, non-aggressive move to your crazy
    brother, who curses you.
You ain't got 30 bayonets
You ain't got swinging flashing fists
You ain't got all that speed.
You've just got a simple place of now
A simple place of appreciative being.
Don't rape the food, don't rape the bean.
You are the food, you are the bean
You are the beautiful pungence of the garlic
You are the slow simple sip of the tea.
You are the warmth of the teacup in the hand
You are the warmth of the tea leaves glowing
You are the warmth of the Sun
You are the simplicity of the Sun
You are the simplicity of the tree
You are the grandeur and simplicity of the Sun and the tree.
You simply can say a simple prayer,
You simply say to all, to everyone and everything that
    nourishes you:
Thank you.

16.

Easing Out of Your Fast

When you start to eat again, you will find that smaller portions are satisfying. A little bit of food can seem like a great sufficiency.

One of the happy results of fasting is bridling of appetite. There is no compulsion to compensate for all the food that wasn't eaten.

After a long fast the palate is restored to pristine purity. It prefers the taste of foods that are simple and whole and natural. It tends to reject processed and fragmented foods, as well as alcohol and tobacco.

There are a few general rules to observe immediately after the fast:

- Do not add salt to your food.
- Continue to drink a lot of water—a quart or more a day.
- Eat slowly and chew carefully. (This is always sound advice for anybody.)

We can benefit from Gandhi's vast experience with fasting. For breaking the long fast, Gandhi cautioned:

> I learned that a man emerging from a long fast should not be in a hurry to regain lost strength and should also put a curb on his appetite. More caution and perhaps more restraint are necessary in breaking a fast than in keeping it.

On breaking even a brief fast, it is important to be cautious about what you eat and how much you eat. To avoid overburdening the digestive system, only small amounts of food should be eaten at any time. Moslems semi-fast religiously—and unhealthily—for a month during the winter; they eat nothing during the day and gorge themselves at night. When I was in Tunisia in January 1975, I was consulted on ways my post-fast program could be introduced into the rites.

In my post-fast program I prescribe a diet that equals in length the number of days of the fast. It is also designed to maintain weight control.

17.

Eating Again

During the first day after your fast

In the morning mix two quarts of water with one quart of orange juice or apricot juice.

Sip two teaspoonfuls of the mixture every five or ten minutes in the first hour after breaking the fast. Sip teaspoonfuls at regular intervals throughout the day, but make sure the concoction lasts until bedtime.

During the second day after a fast of two days or longer

The diet consists of a quart of undiluted orange juice or undiluted apricot juice and at least one quart of water.

Drink four ounces of the juice at two-hour intervals. Drink the water in any amounts and whenever you wish.

(The new ingredient in the refeeding diet today is the undiluted fruit juice.)

During the third day after a fast of three days or longer

Drink one quart of undiluted orange juice or undiluted apricot juice—four ounces at a time at two-hour intervals.

Drink one quart of water in any amount and whenever you wish.

Mix one grated apple in two cups of plain yogurt. Divide the combination into five equal "meals." Have a meal every three hours.

(The addition to the diet today is the combination of the grated apple and the yogurt.)

During the fourth day after a fast of four days or longer

Drink one quart of undiluted orange juice or undiluted apricot juice—four ounces at a time at two-hour intervals.

Drink one quart of water in any amount and whenever you wish.

Mix one grated apple, one grated carrot, and two cups of plain yogurt. Divide the combination into five equal meals. Have a meal every three hours.

(The addition to the diet is the grated carrot.)

During the fifth day after a fast of five days or longer

Drink one quart of undiluted orange juice or undiluted apricot juice—four ounces at a time at two-hour intervals.

Drink one quart of water in any amount and whenever you wish.

Mix one grated apple, one grated carrot, one teaspoon of honey, one teaspoon of lemon juice, and two cups of plain yogurt. Divide the combination into five equal meals. Have a meal every three hours.

In addition, eat two slices of zwieback or melba toast, either with one of the meals or as a snack between meals.

(The additions to the diet today are honey, lemon juice, and either zwieback or melba toast.)

During the sixth day after a fast of six days or longer

Drink one quart of undiluted orange juice or undiluted apricot juice—four ounces at a time at two-hour intervals.

Drink one quart of water in any amount and whenever you wish.

Mix one grated apple, one grated carrot, one teaspoon of honey, one teaspoon of lemon juice, and two cups of plain yogurt. Divide the combination into *four* equal meals. Have a meal every *four* hours.

You may also have whenever you wish two slices of zwieback or melba toast and four ground walnuts.

(The new ingredients in the refeeding diet today are the four ground walnuts. Also, there are four meals instead of five.)

During the seventh day after a fast of seven days or longer

Drink one quart of undiluted orange juice or undiluted apricot juice—four ounces at a time at two-hour intervals.

Drink one quart of water in any amount and whenever you wish.

Mix one grated apple, one grated carrot, one teaspoon of honey, one teaspoon of lemon juice, and two cups of plain yogurt. Divide the combination into four equal meals. Have a meal every four hours.

You may also have whenever you wish two slices of zwieback or melba toast, four ground walnuts, a cup of cooked cereal with milk (do not add salt), and one slice of brown bread (pumpernickel).

(The additions to the diet today are the cereal and the brown bread.)

During the eighth, ninth, and tenth days after a fast of such lengths

The same as the seventh day.

During the eleventh day after a fast of eleven days or longer

Drink one quart of undiluted orange juice or undiluted apricot juice—four ounces at a time at two-hour intervals.

Drink one quart of water in any amount and whenever you wish.

Mix one grated apple, one grated carrot, one teaspoon of honey, one teaspoon of lemon juice, and two cups of plain yogurt. Divide the combination into four equal meals. Have a meal every four hours.

You may also have whenever you wish two slices of zwieback or melba toast, four ground walnuts, a serving of cooked cereal (a cup or less) with milk (do not add salt), and one slice of brown bread. In addition, at mealtime or between meals, you may have an eight-ounce serving of cottage cheese topped with a tablespoon of sour cream.

(The additions to the diet today are the cottage cheese and sour cream.)

During the twelfth day after a fast of twelve days or longer

Drink one quart of undiluted orange juice or undiluted apricot juice—four ounces at a time at two-hour intervals.

Drink one quart of water in any amount and whenever you wish.

Mix one grated apple, one grated carrot, one teaspoon of honey, one teaspoon of lemon juice, and two cups of plain yogurt. Divide the combination into four equal meals. Have a meal every four hours.

You may also have whenever you wish two slices of zwieback or melba toast, four ground walnuts, a serving of cooked cereal (a cup or less) with milk (do not add salt), one slice of brown bread, and one eight-ounce serving of cottage cheese topped with a tablespoon of sour cream.

In addition, you may have with one of your meals, or as a separate meal, two potatoes pureed with milk and one teaspoon of butter (but again no salt).

(The addition to the diet today is the pureed potatoes.)

If you fast beyond twelve days

Continue the regimen of the twelfth day for as many additional days as are necessary. For instance, if you fasted for seventeen days, you should adhere to the diet of the twelfth day for five more days.

When you go off the refeeding program, you may wish to initiate a diet based chiefly on vegetables, fruits, nuts and dairy products. The daily fare can be supplemented with a multiple vitamin tablet. Talk it over with your doctor. In any case, get adequate protein.

18.
Keeping Weight Off

"When I start eating again, won't I just gain back all the weight I lost?"

From my observations I would say that the chances are much better for permanent weight-control after fasting than after any diet whatsoever.

A posthospitalization questionnaire was sent to 709 obese individuals who had fasted at the University of Pennsylvania hospital, whose pioneer fasting program was supervised by Dr. Garfield G. Duncan. Of the 50 percent who responded, approximately 46 percent had continued to lose some weight, and 21 percent had remained at the reduced level at which they had completed their fast. In another study, Dr. E. J. Drenick, another fasting pioneer, in California, learned that 37 of 57 patients had continued to lose weight or to maintain their reduced level two years after a fast.

When anyone abstains totally from food, profound changes take place. These changes revise attitudes about food and put appetite into alignment with the body's real needs for energy.

After the fast, a few pounds may come back. This does not necessarily mean you are eating too much. The sodium content in food causes the body to retain fluid, which shows up as weight on the scales.

A fast of a day or two should correct any slight gains in weight, and in fact could lead to lower weight plateaus.

After the initial fast, the average woman can lose an

additional 1½ to 2½ pounds every week on a daily diet of 1300 to 1500 calories. The average man can lose the same amount with the more liberal daily ration of 1500 to 1900 calories.

19.

Fasting Again

"When can I fast again?"

You can always fast for one or two days a week.

Or you may prefer an occasional three-to-five-day fast.

If you have recently completed a fast of 25 days or longer, you should wait six months before repeating it, and then only in a medical setting of course.

Whether you fast a day or three days or five days at a time, the total in any month should not exceed 10 days *if you fast on a regular basis.*

You must never go below the minimum level of weight your doctor recommends.

20.

Longer Fasts

If you are fasting for a week or longer:
- Keep in touch with your doctor.
- Drink at least two quarts of water every day.
- Exercise as much as you can.
- Do not take medication or pills of any kind without your doctor's approval. (During a fast of a few days you may continue with vitamins and minerals.)
- Keep warm.
- Get plenty of fresh air.
- Rest out-of-doors if possible.
- Sunbathe in the morning when direct and prolonged exposure to the Sun is not as dangerous as later in the day (a sensible health measure at any time).
- Do not drink anything except water. No coffee, no tea, no diluted juices, no non-caloric soft drinks, and certainly no alcohol.
- Do not smoke.
- Shower or bathe frequently. (This is hygienically a good idea because the body rids itself of toxins through the skin. To stimulate the skin use a rough, pliable straw mitt as a wash cloth.)
- Avoid hot baths and saunas.
- Be careful of sudden movement; lowered blood pressure can make you dizzy.
- Do not take diuretics.

Opinion is mixed on the subject of car-driving during a long fast. Fasting can lead to euphoria, even to a slight sense of intoxication—conditions unfavorable to safe driving. I do not believe there is any rigid rule to be laid down on the subject. The best guide to whether you should drive is simply how you feel.

(Before starting a long fast, as before starting any long-term weight-reducing diet, it is advisable to have a medical examination that includes a liver profile and an electrocardiogram.)

The dos and don'ts of the longer fast—for best results—are also applicable to the shorter fast, of course; most of them make excellent sense even when you are not fasting.

21.

Breaking the Longer Fast

The return of appetite and the appearance of a clean tongue, fresh mouth odor, and clear urine are sure signs that you have completed your long fast and it is time to start eating again.

These manifestations usually appear around the 25th day of a long fast. They can appear earlier.

Certain symptoms indicate that metabolism is not functioning properly, and they, too, make it imperative for your doctor to end the fast. These symptoms include:

• Persistence of hunger beyond the fourth day (the reason could be an overabundance of insulin) or the unexpected reappearance of appetite.

• An abnormal cardiac rhythm or persistent rapid pulse beat.

• Gastric or intestinal spasm or symptoms of a surgical abdomen. (If the spasm is functional, medications can be given by a doctor and the fast continued.)

• Cardiac asthma.

• Prolonged periods of nausea or vomiting, headaches, dizziness, or weakness.

• A marked fall in plasma and extracellular fluid volume, resulting in varying degrees of postural hypotension. (Your doctor can retard fluid loss with a daily gram of bicarbonate of soda.)

Your doctor may advise you that there is no need to break the fast if you catch a cold or get an upper respiratory infection. In fact, you might get rid of such an illness quicker if you stay on the fast.

22.

Side Effects Can Be Healthy Signs

At the beginning of a fast you may experience some unpleasant side effects such as headaches, nausea, or dizziness.

These should be no cause for alarm or discouragement. They are usually transitory. If they do not disappear after a couple of days, consult your doctor.

These effects are, in fact, healthy signs. They are indications that the body is ridding itself of waste materials. They are a step on the way to feeling really well both physically and mentally.

Do not worry if there *isn't* even a moment of unpleasantness or discomfort; the purification of the system is still going on. I have rarely had a nauseous patient, though nausea is considered normal in the "getting better" process.

A great many people sail through even lengthy fasts without feeling a moment of discomfort. I have never had a moment of discomfort; my coauthor Eugene Boe has fasted frequently and for varying lengths of time and has never had a moment of discomfort. *Attitude does help.*

Gnawing in the stomach is common on the first two to three days of a fast. Remember: It is not a hunger "pang." Nor is it a distress signal. It is simply the alimentary tract accommodating itself to a reduced work load.

The best way to cope with sensations of hunger— those gnawing feelings in the stomach—is to drink water more frequently.

It is amazing how quickly and well a few sips of water can satisfy what feels like a ravenous appetite.

In the first week of the fast your tongue will become coated. The tongue is part of the elimination system. You may have bad breath, but remember, it is a healthy sign. Your tongue is a "mirror" that reflects the amount of waste matter being eliminated.

You may rinse your mouth with warm water, and you may brush your teeth and tongue very gently with a soft toothbrush. Do not use a mouthwash. No artificial colors, flavors or sweeteners should be used during a fast—mouthwashes contain all of these substances. Toothpastes contain artificial flavors and also should be avoided.

Natural disappearance of the tongue coating and of the acetone odor of the breath precede the return of appetite and are signs that the fast should be broken. The mouth then has a pleasant, fresh taste and the breath smells fresh.

23.
A Brief History of Fasting

Early Egyptians believed that the basis for preserving good health and youthfulness was a fast of three days a month. It apparently had beneficial results. The historian Herodotus described the Egyptians as an extremely healthy people.

The Protean figures in ancient Greece fasted. Pythagoras, the mathematician, was convinced that fasting aided the mental processes. He fasted 40 days at a time, and urged his students to do the same. Socrates and Plato enjoyed ten-day fasts. They claimed that fasting helped them to achieve the ultimate in cerebral functioning. Plutarch said: "Instead of using medicine, better fast today."

Spartans were raised to be spartan in their eating habits.

Aurelius Celsus fasted to treat his jaundice and epilepsy. The Arab physician Avicenna prescribed fasting for all ailments.

In ancient Japan a man could humiliate an enemy by camping on his doorstep and refusing to eat. Centuries ago in India prisoners resorted to fasting to soften their treatment by jailers. In both countries fasting is still commonplace, though the motivations have changed.

The ancient Hebrews fasted in mourning and in times of peril. They also fasted to express gratitude to God for His compassion in sparing them punishment, danger, or calamity. The Day of Atonement is still a day of fasting in the Hebrew calendar.

The Zends went without food every fifth day, the

Syrians every seventh, and the Mongolians every tenth.

Druid priests endured prolonged fasting before initiation into the mysteries of their cult.

Borrowing from the examples of Christ and the Apostles, the earliest Christians fasted on Wednesdays and Fridays—and, later, Saturdays.

Christians also turned to fasting in penance for any misfortune that befell them. In times of general disaster, a fast day was often proclaimed by a bishop.

The linking of almsgiving with fasting started through the custom of turning over to the poor those provisions saved on fast days.

It was once widely believed that demons entered the body of a man when he ate. To commune with God man first had to exorcise the demons and purify himself. He did this by abstaining from food. According to the Book of Matthew, "They goeth not out save by prayer and fasting."

In A.D. 110 Polycarp urged fasting as a way of warding off temptation and lust.

Fasting among Christians symbolized the suffering of Christ. Around the beginning of the fourth century, a time of great persecution, the Lenten fast was introduced. The 40-day abstention was meant to emulate the earlier examples of Moses, Jesus, and Elijah.

Arab physicians of the 10th and 11th centuries prescribed three-week fasts as a cure for syphilis and smallpox. During Napoleon's occupation of Egypt, hospitals used fasting as a treatment for venereal disease.

Ludwig Carnaro, a Venetian in the Renaissance, proposed fasting as the palliative for over-indulgence in the pleasures of food and drink. A year of strict dieting and occasional fasts restored his own health after it had been ravaged by years of dissipation. At the salty old age of 83 Carnaro wrote treatises that celebrated the benefits of fasting:

> Poor, unfortunate Italy! Don't you see that gluttony leads to the death of your citizens, many more deaths than even a worldwide plague or a worldwide war? These disgraceful banquets which are now so popular have results equal to those of the most violent battles.

We must . . . eat only as much as is absolutely necessary for proper functioning of our body and use common sense. Any excess food gives us only the sensory
pleasure of the moment but in the end we have to
pay the consequences of sickness and sometimes even
death.

In England a Dr. Chain (1671–1743) cured himself
of the excesses of food and drink through fasting. He
often prescribed his own "medicine": "I do not know
how it is in other countries," Dr. Chain wrote, "but
we Protestants do not consider . . . excess eating injurious. People look down on friends who are not able
to stuff themselves at every meal. Doctors do not realize
that they should be held responsible before society, their
patients, and even the Creator for propagating excess
eating and thus cutting short the lives of many of their
patients."

Frederick Hoffman (1660–1742), a German, found
fasting to be helpful in treating epilepsy, ulcers, plethora,
cataracts, scurvy, and malignant ulcers. "In any illness,"
he declared, "it is best for the patient not to eat anything."

Russians came to a similar conclusion in the 18th
and 19th centuries. In his *Report of Fasting as Prevention of Illness,* published in 1769, the University of
Moscow's Professor Peter Veniaminov advised that it
was best to stop eating completely during illness. "It
gives the stomach a rest period, enabling the patient to
digest properly when he recovers and starts to eat
again."

B. G. Spassky, also of the University of Moscow, later
reported success in treating intermittent fever with fasting. He said that it allows the growing processes in the
body to take place without interference and "is thus a
perfect remedy for chronic ailments."

Still another Russian, a 19th-century physician, Dr.
Zealand by name, reported that fasting affected a patient's nervous system and his general health, digestion,
and blood—all positively. "Fasting allows the body to
rest and resume its normal activity with renewed
strength," Dr. Zealand wrote.

Dating back to the Plymouth Colony, days of fasting were designated in colonial New England as ways of holding at bay a multitude of catastrophes: droughts, insect plagues, epidemic diseases, Indian wars, earthquakes and food shortages. Fast days were observed as scrupulously as the Puritan sabbath itself.

North American Indians held fasting in high esteem. Among the Algonquins the ability to forgo food for long periods of time was envied and admired as evidence of powers of endurance and fortitude. Hunters fasted before setting out for the kill.

Interest in fasting as a therapeutic tool began in this country during the last century. "Although beginning my practice in fog-covered medical superstition," Dr. Edward Dewey wrote a century ago, "I came to the conclusion that only nature can practice medicine." He prescribed fasting for stomach and intestinal disorders, obesity, dropsy, various infections and inflammations, elimination of physical weakness and flabbiness, and improvement of morale. It was his opinion that it is rest, not food, that repairs the nervous system and that eating causes as much tension as does work.

"I contend that during illness feeding becomes a burden to the sick," Dr. Dewey also wrote. "It uses energy that otherwise would be used to fight the illness."

The dramatic "hunger strike"—fasting in public—to protest political and social injustices is an age-old stratagem. It draws attention to a cause, and often results in remedial action. A fast carried on too long will cross the line into starvation, and few of the powers-that-be want to jeopardize their strength by creating martyrs.

A celebrated fast in Britain in the early 1900s was undertaken by a member of Mrs. Emmeline Pankhurst's Women's Social and Political Union. Marion Wallace Dunlop, a suffragette, fasted to protest a month's jail sentence for inscribing on the wall of the House of Commons a clause from the U.S. Bill of Rights. Hundreds of militant women—and some sympathetic males —joined Ms. Dunlop in the fast and were promptly jailed. In a typical British class action, they all then fasted in objection to their status as ordinary convicts.

Parliament passed a "cat and mouse" act, permitting hunger strikers judged to be in danger of collapse to leave prison for a few days. Once out, most of the fasters discreetly "got lost" and stayed lost. (Women got the vote in 1918.)

In modern times it was Gandhi who popularized fasting as a means of dramatizing a cause. Again it was British law that was successfully challenged.

A Sikh leader fasted for 47 days to persuade the government to establish a separate, Punjab-speaking state. A yogi and a swami fasted to gain assurance that the Punjab state would *not* be partitioned.

The renowned British biologist J. B. S. Haldane fasted for one week, when living in Calcutta, in protest of the U.S. Information Agency's "anti-scientific and anti-Indian activities."

Bridget Rose Dugdale, accused mastermind in the theft of $20-million worth of art treasures for Irish terrorists, fasted to force the transfer of four convicted terrorists from British to Irish jails.

In Russia the imprisoned Vladimir Bukovsky fasted when he was confined to solitary on charges of anti-Soviet agitation; he was joined in the fast by other prisoners. At Radcliffe College students fasted to protest housing rules.

24.

A Noble Tradition

Since the dawn of religion, fasting has been a ritual.

Demons were commonly thought to enter into the body of man through food. "He who wishes to have intercourse with God must thus be abstemious in order to become a pure vessel of the Spirit."

There are no less than 74 references to fasting in the Old and New Testaments. Here are just a few of them:

Moses fasted for 40 days and 40 nights before he received the Ten Commandments on Mount Sinai.

Elijah fasted for 40 days and 40 nights before reaching the Mount of God.

Daniel fasted before receiving divine revelation.

The Book of Chronicles declares that greater closeness with God was obtained throughout Judea by a declaration of a national fast.

Jesus fasted for 40 days and 40 nights.

"When you fast," the Book of Matthew states, "do not look dismal, like the hypocrites." And: "Be honest, be sincere. Fast for honest and truthful purposes."

The disciples of Eastern mysticism embrace fasting with fervor. Yogis fast in the hope of achieving new mystical revelations. In Japan the disciples of Buddha fast as an exercise in asceticism. Dr. Imamura Motoo, who has supervised many fasts, wrote: "Religious ascetics, who led their lives abstaining from food, came to the conclusion that fasting improved not only their spiritual state, but also their physical condition, and through fasting many diseases could be cured."

Edward J. Farrell, a writer specializing in books on

religion, has described fasting as a "religious value . . . having a marvelous resiliency and life span co-extensive with humanity itself. What the parents throw away as useless, the children bring back as new-found treasures. What one generation discards, the next generation unearths and enshrines . . . man should look to his inner resources, his unused power, his hidden self . . . [but] the consumer society generates its antithesis . . . fasting precedes the rebirth of nature, sowing and harvesting . . ."

Russian icon painters would fast at least one day before painting—to get ready, to get in the mood.

Pope Paul VI has said fasting would be a symbolic expression of solidarity with the world's poor. "Man must through fasting dispose himself even materially to allowing his neighbor to share his property in spite of the claims of self-love."

25.

Fasting, Feasting, and Fat

Henry VIII may have set a good table, but at the same time he set a bad example. To this day his name conjures up images of unrestrained gluttony.

The future King George IV, who was one of Henry's successors, also lived high off the hog. In 1817 he hosted a dinner party at Brighton Pavilion, with the famous chef Marie Antoine Carême presiding over this menu:

Consommé Madeira, with foie gras, truffles, mushrooms
River trout with tomato and garlic sauce
Poached turbot in lobster sauce
Eel festooned with cocks' combs
Braised goose
Salmon steak with herbs, butter, and anchovies
Sauteed pheasant segments with truffles
Breast of young wild rabbits
Stuffed partridges in aspic
Meadow larks en terrine with creamed chicken liver
    encased in oven-toasted bread

And these were only the appetizers!

Let George eat it. As delectable as such a Brobdingnagian feast must have been, it was hardly the kind of repast to promote good health and vigor.

Surely no one these days is eating like Henry or George. We are not eating as much as even our grandparents did, but—unlike our grandparents—we are overweight.

Most of us know the reason why we are overweight. We are taking in more fuel than we are burning up. We live in an automated, push-button culture that's made us soft, flabby, and lazy. But too many of us are eating as if we were gandy dancers, lumberjacks, or farmhands; we are also feeding on junk foods that supply us with a diet rich in "empty calories."

Anyone who is 30 pounds overweight is in effect carrying around a 30-pound bag everywhere he goes. Obesity is defined as being 20 percent over one's preferred weight—and more than 45-million Americans *fall* into this category, as we noted earlier.

Here are a few random observations on fat:

• In a study of obesity among adolescents, Dr. Jean Mayer found that fat girls were burning up far fewer calories than lean girls.

• Dr. Mayer also has reported: "In colleges where acceptance was conditioned on a personal interview, the obese girls had only one-third as good a chance of being accepted as their normal-weight classmates; the obese boys had half as good a chance."

• Dr. Walter Lyon Bloom observed that lean people average one hour a day less in bed and spend 23 percent more time on their feet than do the obese.

• Few fat people live out their biblical allotment of threescore and ten years. The only common cause of death that does not take the fat earlier than the lean is suicide.

• Being fat—as well as increasing the risk of heart attacks, high blood pressure, and diabetes—raises the possibility of having gallstones and gallbladder disorders, and makes one more prone to accidents.

• The fat may not know when they are hungry. People who are not overweight tend to eat only when they *are* hungry. ("If it is six o'clock, I am hungry and must have my dinner," the fat person reasons, even though it is only 4:00 P.M. and some trickster has set the hands of the clock ahead.)

• "Nobody loves a fat man, especially not himself," Dr. Theodore Rubin observed in Consumer Guide's *Rating the Diets.* "If he didn't need love so much, he probably would not be fat in the first place."

• "The fat," according to one well-publicized study, think of themselves as generally "unhappy, nervous, tense, and dissatisfied."

• Fat people are likely to try to eat their way out of trouble. As children, they may not have learned to tell the difference between hunger and fear. As adults, they do not know whether they are hungry or just distraught.

• Seating in public places is almost always an irksome problem for the fat, one often caused, noted "the unstylishly stout" Richard F. Shepard in *The New York Times,* by restrictive armrests or limited leg room.

• It is financially punitive to be fat. Obese people pay higher insurance premiums, and the cost for treating ailments induced by obesity can be prohibitive. A survey of 15,000 executives revealed that fat bosses receive less pay than lean bosses. Policemen and firemen have been ordered to trim down or face dismissal—shape up or ship out.

• The overweight are often undernourished. Poor diets, lacking in essential nutrients, are cheaper, and they are usually fat-making. (This explains why there are more poor fat people than rich fat people.)

• We may be born with genes that program us to be fat.

• Overfeeding an infant during the first six months of its life increases the fat in every body cell. This can lead to a life-long fate of being fat.

• Fat parents who want their fat children to lose weight would do well to get *themselves* in shape first. Setting an example is more persuasive than words— always.

26.

Fasting Away from Home

Since the mid-19th century, in clinics and sanitoriums in Switzerland, France, Russia, India, and Germany, fasting has been used in the treatment of patients suffering from metabolic disorders, allergic diseases, skin disorders, arthritis, asthma, ulcerative colitis, cardiovascular complaints, and grand mal epilepsy.

The fasting treatment has also had enthusiastic supporters in the United States—exclusive of the medical profession. (In spite of the overwhelming data—see the Bibliography—most of my colleagues are still not seriously interested in exploring its potentials.)

Lack of encouragement from the medical profession notwithstanding, fasting is entering the mainstream of American life. Thousands of us are making a place for it in our busy lives. With rising levels of health consciousness, more and more of us are choosing to take a vacation from eating when we take our vacation from work, a time that traditionally was devoted to promiscuous gorging.

A fasting vacation is best accomplished under supervision and in the company of others. There are a number of spas and retreats that offer fasting as part of a general health-building regimen. Their attractions usually include tranquil settings, sunshine, facilities for exercise, and carefully supervised diets of natural foods.

Bibliography

Adler, Nathan. "Paris Had Its Hippies in the 1830s: They Drove the Establishment Mad," *Perspectives on Drugs and Drug Use,* no. 3 (1970): 55–59.

Altman, Lawrence K. "Soft Water Tied to Heart Attacks," *New York Times,* June 3, 1974.

America. "To Fast or Not to Fast," March 31, 1962: 849.

American Heart Association. "Diet and Coronary Heart Disease" (1973).

Andersen, Mogens. "Fasting Electrocardiogram," *ACTA Medica Scandinavica,* 187 (1970).

——. Letter to Jerome Agel, June 25, 1974.

Aoki, Thomas T., et al. "Hormonal Regulation of Glutamine Metabolism in Fasting Man," *Advances in Enzyme Regulation* 10 (1972):145–51.

Azar, Gordon and Bloom, Walter. "Ketones, Nonesterified Fatty Acids, and Nitrogen Excretion," *Archives of Internal Medicine* 112, no. 3 (1963):343.

Babayanz, R. "'Natural Stimulator," *Nediela (Izvestia),* April 5, 1970.

Babayanz, R., et al. "The Experience of Using Fasting-Diet Therapy in Dermatology," *Vestnik Dermatalogic i Venerologic* 7, no. 8 (1972).

Baird, I. MacLean. Letter to Jerome Agel, June 10, 1974.

Baird, I. MacLean and Howard, Alan N. "Obesity: Medical and Scientific Aspects," *Proceedings of the First Symposium of The Obesity Association of Great Britain,* London (1968).

Ball, Michael F. "Tissue Change During Intermittent Starvation and Caloric Restriction as Treatment for Severe Obesity," *Archives of Internal Medicine* 125 (1970):62–68.

Ballantyne, D. A. Letter to Editor, *British Medical Journal,* Aug. 7, 1971: 370.

——. Letter to Jerome Agel, June 15, 1974.

Barkas, Janet. *The Vegetable Passion: A History of the Vege-*

127

tarian State of Mind (New York: Scribner's, 1975).

Baruh, Selum, et al. "Fasting Hypoglycemia," *Medical Clinics of North America* 57, no. 6 (1973).

Benedict, Ruth Fulton. "The Vision in Plains Culture," *American Anthropologist* 24 (1922):1–22.

Better Homes & Gardens. "Fasting," Feb. 1961.

Bieler, Henry G. *Food Is Your Best Medicine* (New York: Random House, 1965).

Bishop, Jerry E. "Cancer vs. What You Eat," *Science Digest,* March 1974: 10–14.

Bloom, Walter. "Fasting as an Introduction to the Treatment of Obesity," *Metabolism* 8 (1959):214–20.

———. "Fasting Ketosis in Obese Men and Women," *Journal of Laboratory and Clinical Medicine* 59 (1962):605–12.

———. "Inhibition of Salt Excretion by Carbohydrate," *Archives of Internal Medicine* 109, no. 1 (1962).

———. "Obesity and Energy Expenditure," *Journal of the Medical Association of Georgia* 56, no. 9 (1967):381–82.

Bloom, Walter and Azar, Gordon. "Changes in Heart Size and Plasma Volume During Fasting," *Metabolism* 15, no. 5 (1966):409–13.

———. "Similarities of Carbohydrate Deficiency and Fasting," *Archives of Internal Medicine* 112, no. 3 (1963):333–43.

Bloom, Walter and Mitchell, William. "Salt Excretion of Fasting Patients," *Archives of Internal Medicine* 106, no. 3 (1960): 321–25.

Bonnet, F., et al. "Free Fatty Acid Pattern in the Plasma of Normal and Obese Children During Fasting and Intravenous Glucose Tolerance Test," *Archives of Int. Physiol. BioChim.* 78, no. 3 (1970): 495–508.

Boulter, Philip R., et al. "Dissociation of the Renin-Aldosterone System and Refractorines to the Sodium-Retaining Action of Mineralocorticoid During Starvation in Man," *Journal of Clinical Endocrinology and Metabolism* 38, no. 2 (1974): 248–54.

Bragg, Paul C. *The Miracle of Fasting* (Santa Ana, Calif.: Health Science, 1973).

Braly, Malcolm. "Terror Stalks the Fat Farm," *Playboy,* Jan. 1974.

Brodsky, Greg. *From Eden to Aquarias: The Book of Natural Healing* (New York: Bantàm Books, 1974).

Brosius, J. M. Report to Jerome Agel, 1974.

Brožek, Josef. "Psychology of Human Starvation and Nutritional Rehabilitation," *Scientific Monthly* 70 (1950):270–74.

Bruce, David L. "Anesthetic Implications of Fasting," *Anesth. Analg.* 50, no. 4 (1971):612–19.

Bruch, Hilde. *Eating Disorders* (New York: Basic Books, 1973).

Brown, David F., et al. "Fasting and Postprandial Serum Triglyceride Levels in Healthy Young Americans," *American Journal of Clinical Nutrition* 13, no. 1 (1963):1–7.

Buchinger, Otto H. F. *Everything You Want to Know About Fasting* (New York: Pyramid Books, 1972).

———. "Über Moderne Heilfasten Juren" ("About Modern Fasting Cures"), Buchinger Clinics (1970).

———. "What 40,000 Fasting Treatments Have Taught Me," Buchinger Clinics.

Buchwald, Art. "The Secret of Dieting," *Food and Fitness.*

Butz, Earl L. Statement by the Secretary of Agriculture Before the Subcommittee on Agricultural Production, Marketing and Stabilization of Prices, U.S. Senate, March 21, 1974.

Cahill, George F., Jr. "How Fasting Works," *New England Journal of Medicine* 282 (1970):668–75.

———. "Physiology of Insulin in Man," *Diabetes* 20, no. 12 (1971):785–99.

Cahill, George F., Jr., et al. "The Consumption of Fuels During Prolonged Starvation," *Advances in Enzyme Regulation* 6 (1967):143–50.

———. "Fat and Nitrogen Metabolism in Fasting Man," *Hormone and Metabolic Research,* Supp. 2 (1970).

———. "Hormone Fuel Interrelationships During Fasting," *Journal of Clinical Investigation* 45, no. 11 (1966):1751–67.

Carlson, A. J. and Hoelzel, F. "The Alleged Disappearance of Hunger During Starvation," *Science* 115 (1952):526–27.

Carlson, Anton J., et al. *Machinery of the Body* (Chicago: University of Chicago Press, 1961).

Cavagnini, F., et al. Letter to Editor, *British Medical Journal,* May 19, 1971: 527.

Chase, Alice. *Nutrition for Health* (West Nyack, N.Y.: Parker Publishing Co., 1970).

Chaussain, J. L. "Glycemic Response to 24 Hour Fast in Normal Children and Children with Ketotic Hypoglycemia," *Journal of Pediatrics* 82, no. 3 (1973):438–43.

Christensen, Niels Juel. "Plasma Norepinephrine and Epinephrine in Untreated Diabetics, During Fasting and After Insulin Administration," *Diabetes* 23, no. 1 (1974).

Christianity Today. "Fasting as Therapy," May 12, 1972: 12.

Claiborne, Craig. "The Cure in Italy: Strict Diet, Plus That Funny Tasting Water," *New York Times,* July 11, 1974.

Clark, Blake. "A Swift, Sure Way to Take Off Weight," *Reader's Digest,* Nov. 1962: 115–18.

Cloud, Wallace. "After the Green Revolution," *Sciences,* Oct. 1973.

Corseri, Gary. "Fast, Fast, Fast!", *The New York Times,* March 12, 1975, Op-Ed page.

Costamaillere, L., et al. "Experience With Diagnosis and Treatment of Fasting Hypoglycemia," *Revista Medica de Chile* 100, no. 6 (1972):656–64.

Cott, Allan. "Controlled Fasting Treatment of Schizophrenia in U.S.S.R.," *Schizophrenia* 3, no. 1 (1971):2–10.

Craddock, Denis. *Obesity and Its Management* (Edinburgh: E. & S. Livingstone, 1969).

Crahay, Roland. "Psychology of Fasting," *Abbottempo* (Chicago: Abbott Laboratories).

Cravario, A., et al. *Report on Fasting of 25 Obese Females.*

Cravetto, C. A. "Metabolic Aspects After Prolonged Fasting in Obese Subjects," *Folia Endocrinologica* 26, no. 2 (1973): 139–52.

Critchfield, Richard. "The Sputtering 'Green Revolution,'" *Nation*, Sept. 10, 1973: 207–11.

Cromey, Robert. "For God's Sake, Fast For Your Own Sake!" *Christian Century*, Feb. 28, 1968: 254.

Cubberly, Peter T., et al. "Lactic Acidosis and Death After The Treatment of Obesity by Fasting," *New England Journal of Medicine* 272, no. 12 (1965):628–30.

Current Literature. "'The Fasting Cure' Found Wanting by a Gastronomic Authority," 51 (1911):163–65.

———. "Table Talk: Concerning Eating and Drinking," 35 (1903):761.

Current Therapy. "Obesity: Method of Walter Lyon Bloom" (1960).

DeVries, Arnold. *Therapeutic Fasting* (Los Angeles: Chandler Book Co., 1963).

Drenick, Ernst J. "Weight Reduction by Prolonged Fasting," *Medical Times* 100, no. 1 (1972):209–30.

Drenick, Ernst J. and Dennin, H. F. "Energy Expenditure in Fasting Obese Men," *Journal of Laboratory and Clinical Medicine* 81, no. 3 (1973):421–30.

Drenick, Ernst J., et al. "Body Potassium Content in Obese Subjects and Potassium Depletion During Prolonged Fasting," *American Journal of Clinical Nutrition* 18, no. 4 (1966): 278–85.

———. "Effect on Hepatic Morphology of Treatment of Obesity by Fasting, Reducing Diets and Small-Bowel Bypass," *New England Journal of Medicine* 282, no. 15 (1970): 829–34.

———. "Magnesium Depletion During Prolonged Fasting of Obese Males," *Journal of Clinical Endocrinology and Metabolism* 29, no. 10 (1969):1341–48.

———. "Prolonged Starvation as Treatment for Severe Obesity," *Journal of the American Medical Association* 187, no. 2 (1964):140–45.

Duncan, Garfield G. "Obesity—Some Consideration of Treatment," *American Journal of Clinical Nutrition* 13 (1963): 199.

Duncan, Garfield G. "Contraindications and Therapeutic Results of Fasting in Obese Patients," *Annals of New York Academy of Sciences* 131, Art. 1 (1965):632–36.

————. "The Control of Obesity by Intermittent Fasts," *Medical Clinics of North America* 48, no. 5 (1964):1359–72.

————. "Correction and Control of Intractable Obesity," *Journal of the American Medical Association* 181, no. 4 (1962):99–102.

————. "Intermittent Fasts in the Correction and Control of Intractable Obesity," *American Journal of the Medical Sciences* 245, no. 5 (1963):515–19.

Duncan, L. J. P., et al. "Phenmetrazine Hydrochloride and Methyl Cellulose in the Treatment of 'Refractory' Obesity," *Lancet* i (1960):1262–65.

Ebony. "Hints on Keeping Slim from Famous Personalities," November 1974.

Edison, Thomas A. "Edison on How to Live Long," *Hearst's Magazine*, 23 (1913): 266–69.

Ehret, Arnold. *Rational Fasting: A Scientific Method of Fasting Your Way to Health* (New York: Benedict Lust Publications, 1971).

Encyclopaedia Britannica, 1973 ed., "Fasting."

Encyclopedia Judaica, 1971 ed., "Fasting and Fast Days," 6:1190–96.

Ende, Norman. "Starvation Studies With Special Reference to Cholesterol," *American Journal of Clinical Nutrition* 11, no. 4 (1962):270–80.

Farrell, Edward J. "The Fast of the Body and the Hunger of the Spirit," *New Catholic World*, March/April 1974: 64–68.

Fernstrom, John D., and Wurtman, Richard J. "Nutrition and the Brain," *Scientific American*, 230, no. 2 (1974): pp. 84–91.

Fioravanti, Robert V. "Seeks Personal Stories on Hypoglycemia," Letter to Editor, *Prevention*, Oct. 1973.

Forbes, Gilbert B. "Weight Loss During Fasting: Implications for the Obese," *American Journal of Clinical Nutrition* 23, no. 9 (1970):1212–19.

Fosburgh, Lacey. "Scientist Fears Wide Food Shortage," *New York Times*, Feb. 28, 1974.

Fox, George. "Wanted: A Science of Nutrition," *Prevention*, May 1974: 59–64.

Fox, J. DeWitt. "Fasting for Fitness," *Life & Health* 80, no. 1 (1965):6–7.

Franklin, Maxine A. and Skoryna, Stanley C. "Studies in Natural Gastric Flora: Survival of Bacteria in Fasting Human Subjects," *Canadian Medical Association Journal* 105 (1971):380–86.

Fredericks, Carlton. "Hotline to Health," *Prevention*, July 1973: 59.

Fredholm, Bertil B. "Effects of Fasting on Adipose Tissue in situ in Young Dogs," *Scandinavian Journal of Clinical and Laboratory Investigation* 31, no. 1 (1973):79–86.

Galloway, John A. "The Effects of Low Doses of Intravenous Proinsulin and Insulin Combination in Normal Fasted Man," *Journal of Laboratory and Clinical Medicine* 78, no. 6 (1972):991–92.

Gamble, J. L., et al. "The Metabolism of Fixed Base During Fasting," *Journal of Biological Chemistry* 57 (1923):633–95.

Gandhi, M. K. *Gandhi's Autobiography* (1954 ed.).

————. "Why I Fasted for Twenty-one Days," *World Tomorrow* 16 (1933):496–97.

Garnett, E. S., et al. "Gross Fragmentation of Cardiac Myofibrils After Therapeutic Starvation for Obesity," *Lancet* i (1969).

Gasner, Douglas Brian. "The Perils of Lead," *World*, Aug. 1, 1972: 52.

Gault, John. "Prolonged Fasting Tested as Schizophrenia Therapy," *Medical Post*, Nov. 16, 1971: 16.

Genuth, Saul M. "Alanine Administration During Prolonged Fasting," *Medical Post*, Nov. 16, 1971.

Gibinski, Kornel. "Starvation Treatment of Obesity," *Polska Tygodnik Lekarski* 24, no. 25 (1969):951–64.

Gilliland, I. C. "Total Fasting in the Treatment of Obesity," *Postgraduate Medical Journal* 44 (1968):507.

Gligore, V. and Fekete, T. "Complete Fasting Diet (0-Calorie diet) in the Treatment of Obesity," *Revue Roumaine d'Endocrinologie* 10, no. 1 (1973):79–84.

Glueck, Grace H. "Fine Art of Fasting," *New York Times Magazine*, Oct. 8, 1961: 106.

Gol, Barbara. "Fasting: A Radical Medical Approach to Weight Loss," *Town & Country*, Jan. 1973: 32.

Goldman, Ronald, et al., "Yom Kippur, Air France, Dormitory Food, and the Eating Behavior of Obese and Normal Persons," *Journal of Personality and Social Psychology* 10, no. 2 (1968):117–23.

Greene, Gael. Letter to Jerome Agel, Dec. 1974.

Gross, Robert R. "In Defense of Fasting: A Rebuttal to Critiques in Playboy Magazine," *Natural Hygienews*, May 1974.

Grosser, Volker, et al. "Tryptophan Loading During Fasting," *Deutsche Gesundheitwesen*, April 4, 1973: 793–98.

Halloran, Richard. "Japanese Long in Jungle in Fine Health," *New York Times*, April 24, 1974.

Halsell, Grace. "Wisdom on the Hoof," *The New York Times*, March 1, 1975.

Harrison, Michael T. "The Long-Term Value of Fasting in the Treatment of Obesity," *Lancet* ii (1966).

Hauck, Charles R. "How to Break the Nutrition Habit," *New York Times*, Feb. 11, 1974.

Havemann, Ernest. "The Wasteful, Phony, Crash Dieting Craze," *Life*, Jan. 19, 1959: 102–106.

Henderson, J. S. "The Modulation in Fasted Hosts of a Tumor's Growth and the Contrasting Stability of Its Intrinsic Grade of Malignancy," *Journal of Pathology* 109, no. 1 (1973).

Hendrikx, A. and De Moor, P. "Metabolic Changes in Obese Patients During Fasting and Refeeding," *ACTA Clinica Belgica* 24, no. 1 (1969):1–16.

Hermann, L. S. and Iversen, M. "Death During Starvation," Letter to the Editor, *Lancet* ii (1968):217.

Hermann, L. S., et al. "Hyperaldosteronism Following Weight Reduction by Complete Fasting" and "Late Results of Weight Reduction by Complete Fasting," *Videnskab Og Praksis*, Jan. 30, 1969.

Hess, John L. "The Unbalanced American's Diet: 20 Partials, Not 'Three Squares'," *The New York Times*, Jan. 3, 1974.

Heyden, Siegfried H. "Now—The Workingman's Diet," *Reader's Digest*, Jan. 1972.

Heyden, Siegfried H., et al. "Body Weight and Cigarette Smoking As Risk Factors," *Archives of Internal Medicine* 128 (1971):915–19.

———. "Diet Treatment of Obese Hypertensives," *Clinical Science and Molecular Medicine* 45 (1973):209s–12s.

———. "Weight and Weight History in Relation to Cerebrovascular and Ischemic Heart Disease," *Archives of Internal Medicine* 128 (1971):956–60.

———. "Weight Reduction in Adolescents," *Nutrition and Metabolism* 15 (1973):295–304.

Hippocrates Health Institute. Letter to Jerome Agel, July 2, 1974.

Hittleman, Richard L. *Weight Control Through Yoga* (New York: Bantam Books, 1971).

Howard, A. N. Letters to Jerome Agel, April 8 and June 4, 1974.

Howard, Jane. "How I Lost 14 Pounds in a Week," *Family Circle*, Oct. 1974.

Hunscher, Martha A. "A Posthospitalization Study of Patients Treated for Obesity by a Total Fast Regimen," *Metabolism* 15, no. 5 (1966):383–93.

Imaichi, Kunitaro, et al. "Plasma Lipid Fatty Acid During Fasting," *American Journal of Clinical Nutrition* 13, no. 4 (1963):226–31.

Independent. "The Fast Cure—For Fasting," 84 (1915):436.

———. "Fasting as a Religious Experience," Editorial, 56 (1904):980–82.

Innes, J. A., et al. "Long-Term Follow-Up of Therapeutic Starvation," *British Medical Journal* 2 (1974):356–59.

Jahn, Mike. "Fasting Is So Spiritual," *Cosmopolitan*, July 1974.

Johnson, Thomas A. "Monsoon Shift Held Threat to World Food Supply," *New York Times*, Jan. 26, 1974.

Journal of the American Medical Association. "Starvation and Obesity." (Editorial), 187, no. 2 (1964):144.

————. "Three Views of the Treatment and Hazards of Obesity," 186, no. 7 (1963):45–50.

Kahan, Alexander. Letter to the Editor, *Lancet* i (1968):1378.

Kalkhoff, R. K. and Kim, H. J. "Metabolic Responses to Fasting and Ethanol Infusion in Obese, Diabetic Subjects," *Diabetes* 22, no. 5 (1973):372–80.

Katz, Sidney. "Metro Man Recovers from Mental Illness by Fasting 28 Days," *Toronto Star*, Aug. 26, 1972.

Klein, Frederick C. "New Techniques Help Pupils Who Can't Grasp Fundamental Concepts," *Wall Street Journal*, Nov. 17, 1970.

Klemesrud, Judy. "A Week at a Health Manor on the Last Resort Diet: Fasting," *New York Times*, Oct. 29, 1974.

Knobe, Bertha Damaris. "Why I Fasted Fifteen Days," *Ladies Home Journal* 29 (1912).

Knudsen, Kermit B. "Porphyria Precipitated by Fasting," *New England Journal of Medicine* 277, no. 7 (1967).

Knutsson, Karl Eric. "Fasting in Ethiopia. An Anthropological and Nutritional Study," *American Journal of Clinical Nutrition* 23, no. 7 (1970):956–69.

Kollar, Edward J. and Atkinson, Roland M. "The Effectiveness of Fasting in the Treatment of Superobesity," *Psychosomatics* 10, no. 2 (1969).

Komarnicka, R. "Treatment of Obesity with Starvation and Low Calorie Diet," *Polska Tygodnik Lekarski* 29, no. 20 (1974):843–45.

Lageder, H., et al. "Absolute Fasting as Therapy in Patients With Diabetes and Hyperlipaemia," *Wiener Klinische Wochenschrift*, March 23, 1973, p. 186.

Laszlo, J. "Changes in the Obese Patient and His Adipose Tissue During Prolonged Starvation," *Southern Medical Journal* 58 (1965):1099–1108.

Lawlor, T. Letter to Editor. *Lancet* i (1969).

Lawlor, T. and Wells, D. G. "Fasting as a Treatment of Obesity," *Postgraduate Medical Journal*, June Suppl., 1971: 452–58.

————. "Metabolic Hazards of Fasting," *American Journal of Clinical Nutrition* 22, no. 8 (1969):1142–49.

Lennox, William G. "A Study of the Retention of Uric Acid During Fasting," *Journal of Biological Chemistry* 66, no. 2 (1925): 521–72.

Lewis, Anthony. "Affluence and Survival II," *New York Times,* April 22, 1974.

Lissner, Will. "Cooke Asks a Fast to Back Africans," *New York Times,* July 6, 1974.

Literary Digest. "The Dangers of Fasting," 101 (1929): 23.

———. "Facts About Fasting," 95 (1927): 26.

———. "Holy Hunger: Tennessee Mountaineer Believes Fasting Was Divine Command," 123 (1937).

———. "Man a Poor Faster," 114 (1932): 18.

———. "The Starvation Cure," 76 (1923): 77.

Living Age. "The Spirit of Fasting," (1910).

Maagoe, H. and Mogensen, E. F. "The Effect of Treatment on Obesity: A Follow-up Investigation of a Material Treated with Complete Starvation," *Danish Medical Bulletin* 17, no. 7 (1970):206–9.

Macadam, Robert F. and Jackson, A. M. Letter to the Editor, *Lancet* i, May 24, 1969.

McCarthy, Colman. "Fasting: Just Another Fad, or Nation's 'Finest Hour,' " Washington Post Service, Dec. 28, 1974.

McCoy, Kathy. "Winning the Weight War," *Teen,* May 1974: 39.

MacCuish, A. C., et al. "Follow-up Study of Refractory Obesity Treated by Fasting," *British Medical Journal* 1, (1968): 91–92.

McGraw, James R. and Fulton, Alvenia M., eds. *Dick Gregory's Natural Diet for Folks Who Eat: Cooking with Mother Nature* (New York: Harper & Row, 1973).

McHarry, Charles. "On the Town," *New York News,* June 8, 1974.

McMillan, Thelma J. "Your Basic Food Needs: Nutrients For Life, Growth," *Yearbook of Agriculture* (1969): 254–59.

Mahler, H. "Better Food for a Healthier World," *World Health,* Feb/March 1974: 3.

Marliss, Errol B., et al. "Glucagon Levels and Metabolic Effects in Fasting Man," *Journal of Clinical Investigation* 49, no. 12 (1970):2256–70.

Mayer, Jean. *Human Nutrition* (Springfield, Ill.: C. C. Thomas, 1972), chap. 36, "Reducing by Total Fasting."

———. "Obese Are Fair Game for Discrimination," *New York News,* Feb. 26, 1975.

———. *Overweight: Causes, Cost, and Control* (Englewood Cliffs, N. J.: Prentice-Hall, 1968: 161–62.

Medical World News. "In Three Months, Even Autistic Children Respond," Sept. 24, 1971.

Middlebury, Maria. "My Week Without Food," *Good Housekeeping* 53 (1911): 202.

Miller, Arthur. "Sakharov, Détente and Liberty," *New York Times,* July 5, 1974.

Morgulis, Sergius. "Fasting and the Healing Art," *Hygeia* 8 (1930):609–13.

Mottram, R. F. and Baker, Patricia G. B. "Metabolism of Exercising and Resting Human Skeletal Muscle in the Post Prandial and Fasting States," *Clinical Science* 44 (1973): 479–91.

Munro, J. F. and Duncan, L. J. P. "Fasting in the Treatment of Obesity," *Practitioner* 208 (1972): 493–98.

Munro, J. F., et al. "Further Experience With Prolonged Therapeutic Starvation in Gross Refractory Obesity," *British Medical Journal* 4 (1970): 712–14.

NBC News. "You're Too Fat," 1974.

New Catholic Encyclopedia, 1967 ed., 5:847–50.

New Schaff-Herzog Encyclopedia of Religious Knowledge, 1967 ed.: 279–84.

New York News. "Fat Bosses Pull In Their Moneybelts," Jan. 2, 1974: 16.

———. "Jaw Lock Ends Lip Service to Diet," Dec. 1, 1973.

———. "The Thin Girl Within the 'Fat' Person Comes Out," April 18, 1974: 91.

New York Post. "Dieting With Taft's Choice," March 5, 1975.

———. "Fasting for a World of Plenty," Nov. 21, 1974: 17.

The New York Times. "Harry Wills Dead," Dec. 22, 1958: 2.

———. "Sakharov Ends 6-Day Fast," July 5, 1974.

———. "Soviet Prisoners Reported Joining Bukovsky in Fast," April 15, 1972.

New Yorker. "Books: From Abalone to Zimmern, Sir Alfred," Nov. 12, 1973.

Newsweek. "Fast, Fast, Fast," April 15, 1963.

———. "Pangs of Conscience, January 20, 1975: 72.

———. "Running Out of Food?" April 1, 1974: 40–41.

———. "Strictly from Hunger," Nov. 22, 1971: 122–24.

Nikolayev, Yuri. Letter to Dr. Allan Cott, May 1974.

Null, Gary and staff. *The Complete Question and Answer Book of General Nutrition* (New York: Dell, 1974).

Nutrition Reviews. "Changes in Liver Histology and Function in Fasted Human Subjects," 25, no. 10 (1967):295–97.

———. "Hunger During Total Starvation Regimen," 25, no. 2 (1967):40–41.

———. "Lipid Accumulation in Heart Muscle During Fasting," 23, no. 1 (1965):14–16.

———."Long-Term Changes in Body Weight Following Complete Fasting for Obesity," 25, no. 6 (1967):168–70.

———. Potassium Supplementation During Fasting for Obesity," 28, no. 7 (1970):177–78.

———. "Salt Supplementation During Fasting in the Cold," 23, no. 2 (1965):45–46.

Oldfield, Josiah. *Fasting for Health and Life* (London, 1924).

Olefsky, Jerrold, et al. "Effects of Weight Reduction on Obesity," *Journal of Clinical Investigation* 53, no. 1 (1974): 64–76.

Owen, Philip and Cahill, George F., Jr., "Metabolic Effects of Exogenous Glucocorticoids in Fasted Man," *Journal of Clinical Investigation* 52 (1973):2596–604.

Owen, Philip, et al. "Brain Metabolism During Fasting," *Journal of Clinical Investigation* 46, no. 10 (1967).

―――. "Liver and Kidney Metabolism During Prolonged Starvation," *Journal of Clinical Investigation* 48 (1969):574.

Pager, Milton and Iampietro, P. F. "The Effect of Prolonged Cold and Starvation and Subsequent Refeeding on Plasma Lipids and Glucose of Normal Men," *Metabolism: Clinical and Experimental* 15, no. 1 (1966):9–16.

Parekh, Manilal C. "Fasting as a Cure for Lynching," *Christian Century, 52* (1935).

Parker, Donal, et al. "Persistence of Rhythmic Human Growth Hormone Release During Sleep in Fasted and Nonisocalorically Fed Normal Subjects," *Metabolism: Clinical and Experimental* 21, no. 3 (1972):241.

Parnell, R. W. "Fragmentation of Cardiac Myofibrils After Therapeutic Starvation," *Lancet* i (1969):1154.

―――. Letter to the Editor, *Lancet* i (1969).

Parrett, O. S. "Fasting," *Life & Health*, April 1965: 24–26.

Patient Care. A Special Issue. "A Practical Approach to Diet Compliance," April 1, 1973.

Peters, G. "Fasting Cures," *Medizinische Klinik* 63, no. 31 (1968):1209–11.

Porter, A. M. W. Letter to the Editor, *Lancet* i (1968): 1378.

Porter, Sylvia. "Staple Inflation," *New York Post,* May 28, 1974.

Prevention. "Fasting Can Control Schizophrenia," Aug. 1971: 197–201.

Punch. Jan. 9, 1974: 46.

Randolph, Theron G. "Food Addiction and Ecologic Mental Illness" (Chicago: Human Ecology Research Foundation, 1971).

―――. "Food Addiction, Obesity and Alcoholism," *International Journal of Social Psychiatry,* Congress issue (1964).

―――. Letter to Jerome Agel, June 14, 1974.

―――. "The Realities of Food Addiction: 1. Description and Recognition; 2. Treatment and Prophylaxis," *Health Views & News,* nos. 10–11 (1971).

Rath, Rathmer and Masek, Josef. "Changes in the Nitrogen Metabolism in Obese Women after Fasting and Refeeding," *Metabolism: Clinical & Experimental* 15, no. 1 (1966):1–8.

Read, Piers Paul. *Alive* (Philadelphia: Lippincott, 1974).

Reed, Roy. "U.S. Fertilizer Shortage Expected to Be Damaging to Many Poorer Nations," *New York Times,* April 4, 1974.

Robbins, William. "U.S. Needy Found Poorer, Hungrier Than 4 Years Ago," *New York Times,* June 20, 1974, p. 1.

Rochlin, Isidore and Edwards, W. L. Jack. "The Misinterpretation of Electrocardiograms with Postprandial T-wave Inversion," *Circulation* 10 (1954):843–49.

Rooth, G. Letters to Jerome Agel, April 30 and June 18, 1974.

Rooth, G. and Carlström, S. "Therapeutic Fasting," *ACTA Medica Scandinavica* 187 (1970):455–63.

Rooth, G. and Ostenson, S. "Acetone Alveolar Air and the Control of Diabetes," *Lancet* ii (1966).

Rooth, G., et al. "Plasma Tocopherol Levels in Therapeutic Starvation," *International Journal of Vitamin & Nutrition Research* 41 (1971):355–59.

Rothenberg, Robert B. *The Fast Diet Book* (New York: Grosset & Dunlap, 1971).

Runcie, J. "Urinary Sodium and Potassium Excretion in Fasting Obese Subjects," *British Medical Journal* 2 (1971):22–25.

Runcie, J. and Hilditch, T. E. "Energy Provision, Tissue Utilization and Weight Loss in Prolonged Starvation," *British Medical Journal,* May 18, 1974: 352–56.

Runcie, J. and Thomson, T. J. "Prolonged Starvation—A Dangerous Procedure?" *British Medical Journal* 3 (1970): 432–35.

————. "Total Fasting, Hyperuricaemia and Gout," *Postgraduate Medical Journal* 45 (1969):251–53.

Schachter, Stanley. "Obesity and Eating," *Science* 161 (1968): 751–56.

Schanche, Don A. "Diet Books That Poison Your Mind and Harm Your Body," *Today's Health* 52, no. 4 (1974): 56–61.

Schloeder, Francis X., and Steinbaugh, Bobby J. "Defect of Urinary Acidification During Fasting," *Metabolism* 15, no. 1 (1966):17–25.

Schmeck, Harold J., Jr. "Alcoholism Cost to Nation Put at $25-Billion a Year," *New York Times,* July 11, 1974: 1.

————. "World Seen Near a Food Disaster," *New York Times,* March 15, 1974.

Schrub, J.-Cl., et al. "Lipid Changes Induced by Fasting in Obese Subjects," *Semaine des Hopitaux* 49, 19 (1973):1349–56.

Science Digest. "Fasting Record," April 1967: 57.

————. "New 'S' Diet," Feb. 1974: 54.

————. "New Slimming Device," Feb. 1974.

Science News. "Famine and the Third World," 105 (May 11, 1974).

————. "High Protein Diet and Cholesterol," 105 (1974):240.

————. "How Do You Taste," 105 (1974): 29.

————. "Why Wives Overeat," 102 (1972).

Science News Letter, "Add Two Pounds Daily," 83 (1963):403.

————. "Body Changes in Fasting," 66 (1946):5.

————. "To Reduce, Fast 10 Days," 82 (1962):4.

Seeger, Murray. "Soviet Cure-All: Eat Nothing for 30 Days," *Los Angeles Times,* April 3, 1972.

Senior, Boris. Editor's Column, *Journal of Pediatrics* 82, no. 3 (1973):555.

Shabad, Theodore. "Russians Advised to Eat 4 Meals a Day," *New York Times,* June 12, 1972.

Shelton, Herbert M. *Facts About Fasting,* Ahimsa Booklet no. 4 (1972).

————. *Fasting Can Save Your Life* (Chicago: Natural Hygiene Press, 1964).

————. *Fasting for Renewal of Life* (Chicago: Natural Hygiene Press, 1974).

Shepard, Richard F., "For the Stylishly Stout, Portly or Just Fat, Life is Not Easy," *The New York Times,* March 3, 1975.

Sherrill, James W. "A Study in Fasting," *Cyclopedia of Medicine* 5 (1932):626–63.

Shigematsu, M. Letter to Jerome Agel, June 5, 1974.

Simonson, Ernst, et al. "The Effect of Meals on the Electrocardiogram in Normal Subjects," *American Heart Journal* 32 (1946):202–14.

Sinclair, Upton. *The Fasting Cure* (Pasadena, Calif.: Sinclair, 1923).

————. "Fasting—the Foe of Sickness," *Cosmopolitan* 50 (1910–11):328–36.

————. "Starving for Health's Sake," *Cosmopolitan* 48 (1910): 739–46.

Sletten, Ivan W., et al. "Total Fasting in Psychiatric Subjects: Psychological, Physiological and Biochemical Changes," *Canadian Psychiatric Association Journal* 12, no. 6 (1967): 553–58.

Snider, Arthur J. "A Fast Way to Lose Weight," *Chicago Daily News Syndicate,* Oct. 1975.

————. "Nature Fights Starvation," *Science Digest,* May 1972: 48–49.

————. "The Progress of Medicine," *Science Digest,* Oct. 1963: 52–53.

————. "The Woman Who Stopped Eating," *Science Digest,* April 1964: 81–83.

Snyder, Camilla. "Gayelord Hauser: On the Move at 80," *New York Times,* March 24, 1974.

Spencer, Herta, et al. "Changes in Metabolism in Obese Persons During Starvation," *American Journal of Medicine* 40 (1966):27–37.

Spencer, I. O. B. "Death During Therapeutic Starvation for Obesity," *Lancet* i (1968):1288–90.

Stahel, Thomas H., S.J. "When You Fast, Do Not Look Dismal," *America,* March 2, 1974: 161.

Stein, Marjorie. "Dieting to Disaster," *Mademoiselle,* Jan. 1974.

Stewart, William K. and Fleming, Laura W. Letter to the Editor, *Lancet,* June 7, 1969.

———. "Relationship Between Plasma and Erythrocyte Magnesium and Potassium Concentrations in Fasting Obese Subjects, *Metabolism: Clinical and Experimental* 22, no. 4 (1973.)

Stunkard, Albert and McLaren-Hume, Mavis. "The Results of Treatment for Obesity," *Archives of Internal Medicine* 103, no. 1 (1959).

Sullivan, Walter. "Monsoon Shift Called Threat to World Food," *New York Times,* Jan. 26, 1974.

Susskind, Charles. *Understanding Technology* (Baltimore: Johns Hopkins University Press, 1973).

Swanson, David W. and Dinello, Frank A. "Follow-up of Patients Starved for Obesity," *Psychosomatic Medicine* 32, no. 2 (1970):209–14.

———. "Severe Obesity as a Habituation Syndrome: Evidence During a Starvation Study," *Archives of General Psychiatry* 22, no. 2 (1970):120–27.

Swendseid, Marian E., et al. "Nitrogen and Weight Losses During Starvation and Realimentation in Obesity," *Journal of the American Dietetic Association* 46 (1965):276–79.

Tallmer, Jerry. "At Home with Lady Jean Campbell," *New York Post,* April 8, 1972.

Taub, Harold J. "Eat Less to Live More," *Prevention,* Oct. 1973.

Taylor, Henry Longstreet, et al. "The Effect of Successive Fasts on the Ability of Men to Withstand Fasting During Hard Work," *American Journal of Physiology* 143, no. 1 (1945): 148–55.

Teltsch, Kathleen. "Peril to 400 Million Is Seen by UNICEF," *New York Times,* May 14, 1974.

Thomson, T. J., et al. "Treament of Obesity by Total Fasting for Up to 249 Days," *Lancet* ii (1966):992-96.

Thurston, Herbert. "Living Without Eating," *Month* 158 (1931):217–28.

Tiengo, A., et al. "Metabolic and Hormonal Patterns After Three Days of Total Fasting in 27 Obese and Non-Obese Subjects," *Israel Journal of Medical Sciences* 8, 6 (1972): 821–22.

Time. "Fasting Is Not Enough," Dec. 9, 1974: 14.

———. "Fat Faddists, Beware," Dec. 16, 1974: 105–106.

———. "The Return of Fasting," Dec. 16, 1974: 86–87.

———. "Hungry Men," Review of *The Biology of Human Starvation,* by Dr. Ancel Keys, June 12, 1950: 46.

Trecker, Barbara. "The Battle Against Weight," part 5, *New York Post*, Jan. 11, 1974: 35.

U.S. News & World Report. "How Safe Is the Food You Eat?" April 8, 1974: 39–42.

Van Horne, Harriet. "Portents of Doom" and "Farmer Brown: R.I.P.," *New York Post*, 1974.

Van Kuren, Susan. "Doctor Warns of Dangers of Food Additives," *Windsor* (Ont.) *Star*, March 12, 1974.

Verdy, Maurice. "BSP Retention During Total Fasting," *Metabolism: Clinical and Experimental* 15, no. 9 (1966).

————. "Effet de la Renutrition au Glucose Après le Jeûne, sur la Bilirubine et la BSP," *Médicale du Canada* 102 (1973):2514–15.

————. "Fasting in Obese Females," *American Journal of Clinical Nutrition* 23, no. 8 (1970):1033–36.

————. "Fasting in Obese Females: 1. A Study of Thyroid Function Tests, Serum Proteins and Electrolytes," *Canadian Medical Association Journal* 98, no. 22 (1968):1031–33.

Verdy, Maurice and Champlain, Jacques. "Fasting in Obese Females: 2. Plasma Renin Activity and Urinary Aldosterone," *Canadian Medical Association Journal* 98, no. 22 (1968): 1034–37.

Verdy, Maurice and Marc-Aurele, J. "Fasting in Obese Females: Plasma Renin After Glucose Refeeding," *Hormone and Metabolic Research* 5, no. 1 (1973):59.

Village Voice. "Scenes: An Interview with Dr. Allan Cott," Aug. 22, 1974.

Von Hoffman, Nicholas. "Why Be Healthy?" *Prevention*, Feb. 1973: 69.

Wade, Carlson. *The Natural Way to Health Through Controlled Fasting* (New York: Arc Books, 1968).

Walczak, Michael and Huemer, Richard P. *Applied Nutrition in Clinical Practice* (New York: Intercontinental Medical Book Corp., 1973).

Webster, P. D., et al. "Effects of Feeding and Fasting on the Pancreas," *Gastroenterology* 62, no. 4 (1972):600–605.

Weinraub, Bernard. "Lag in Fertilizer Threatens India," *New York Times*, April 4, 1974.

Weinsier, Roland L. "Fasting: A Review with Emphasis on the Electrolytes," *American Journal of Medicine* 50, no. 2 (1971):233–40.

Westermarck, Edward. "The Principles of Fasting," *Folk-Lore* 18, no. 4 (1907):391–422.

Windmueller, H. G. "Elevated Riboflavin Levels in Urine of Fasting Human Subjects," *American Journal of Clinical Nutrition* 15, no. 2 (1964).

Winter, Ruth. "Are you a 'Yo-Yo' Dieter?" *Science Digest*, May 1974: 36–40.

Woodham-Smith, Cecil. *The Great Hunger: Ireland 1845–184'*
(New York: Harper & Row, 1962).
────. *Queen Victoria* (New York: Dell, 1974).
Young, Vernon R. and Scrimshaw, Nevin S. "The Physiology
of Starvation," *Scientific American* 225, no. 4 (1971): 14–
21.
Zborowski, Mark and Herzog, Elizabeth. *Life Is with People:
The Culture of the Shtetl* (New York: Schocken Books,
1965).

BONUS BOOK
AT NO EXTRA CHARGE

The bestselling sequel

FASTING
AS A WAY OF LIFE

by Allan Cott, M.D.

with Jerome Agel
and Eugene Boe

produced by Jerome Agel

Contents

Note

Fasting has been a way of life, voluntarily or involuntarily, since primordial man first began to scrounge for food and to try to placate an avenging divine power.

Modern man foregoes food principally to lose weight the quickest and easiest way; to give the body a rest; to feel better physically and mentally; and to save money on food bills. But there are more than a score of other reasons to fast.

Because nature takes good care of the body during a fast, the person in average good health can fast safely for up to four weeks. (A long fast should be done only under the direct supervision of a doctor experienced in the fasting procedure.)

The applications of fasting are proliferating in our busy, stressful, consciousness-expanding, health-seeking society. Employees of an enlightened manufacturer in the Midwest fast for "a sense of renewal." Star athletes train on "the ultimate diet." Hundreds of thousands of Americans—from every walk of life—altruistically celebrate the Thursday before Thanksgiving as a national fast day.

Numerous applications of fasting are reported here, as are healthier eating regimens and medical-research discoveries. There is now reason to believe that the fasted body will not "accept" in quantity alcohol, nicotine, drugs, or other toxic substances.

People planning to fast on their own should find this book informative and supportive. But *Fasting as a Way of Life* is not intended to take the place of professional care or consultation. As we strongly emphasized in *Fasting: The Ultimate Diet,* a person planning to fast even for a day should—as with any diet—first consult her or his doctor. Anyone undertaking a longer fast should be under the doctor's close supervision throughout the fast and for the entire period of adjustment after the fast. Though fasting can be therapeutic, the emphasis in this book is principally on fasting as a way of life for people in at least average good health.

—Allan Cott, M.D.

Fasting
as a Way of Life

1.
Fear of Fasting

*"I feel like a wisp of cloud, full of light and energy.
It's a magical rest for my whole system."*

*"I've never felt so well, I've never been so thin, I've
never had so much free time."*

"I now have greater respect for my body's intelligence and capability. Fasting is a marvelous life-lesson."

*"Once I got rid of the cultural hang-up that I've got
to eat all the time, fasting was a snap!"*

These are typical expressions reflecting the ease,
comfort, and even exhilaration of the fasting experience.

Yet fasting remains controversial. There are still
those whose attitudes toward going without food for
even one day are frozen in fear and ignorance. "It's
too dangerous," they say. Or "I'd pass out if I didn't
eat 'three squares' a day." Or "I'm afraid I'd starve to
death."

An ironic consequence of the popularity of my first
book, *Fasting: The Ultimate Diet,* was that it revived
some of those fears and prejudices, though I was confident my extensive documentation demonstrated them
to be unfounded.

Incredibly, some doctors still believe it is "dangerous" for anyone to abstain from a single meal, and they
resurrect the fallacies when asked about "the ultimate
diet." Man is the only "animal" who persists in eating

or is forced to eat even when he is sick, though he may have no appetite and food makes him nauseous.

(To some Americans, fasting may be idiosyncratic precisely because we are an overabundant society producing more foodstuffs than we need to consume.)

If disparaging doctors would take the time to examine the evidence dispassionately, they would finally stop warning of "dangers" that simply do not exist for most people. They owe it to their patients to become more knowledgeable because this remarkable discipline has stood the test of time—at least five thousand years.

It apparently needs to be said over and over again: "Fasting is *not* starving, fasting is *not* starving, fasting is *not* starving. . . ."

The body has in reserve at least *a month's* supply of food. It nourishes itself during a fast as if it were continuing to receive food. When this stockpile is consumed, the body signals by the return of appetite that it is time to start the refeeding program.

Dr. George F. Cahill, Jr., of the Harvard School of Medicine, put this crucial fact in a nutshell: "Man's *survival* is predicated upon a remarkable ability to conserve the relatively limited body protein stores while utilizing fat as the primary energy-producing food."

I know many grossly overweight people who still think of fasting as starving. They shy away from the idea of even a brief fast, even though they would benefit most from "the ultimate diet."

I remind these people that in many controlled experiments here and abroad it has been documented that the obese tolerate fasting far better than any other weight-reducing regimen. Such men and women find they can go long periods without feeling hungry, for the fasting body *automatically* dims the memory of food and normalizes metabolism. The rate of weight loss is also extremely supportive of self-esteem, which had diminished with each prior unsuccessful dieting experience.

(The food editor of a metropolitan newspaper, by her own admission, weighed 60 pounds more than she should. But she believed she couldn't consider fasting for even a day because she'd "starve to death." Also, she had been told by her doctor that anyone who fasts must be "insane.")

The body does not consume itself in any vital way even during an extended fast. This is the principal difference between the life-enhancing act of fasting and the self-destructive act of starving. But misleading books about fasting are still being published; they use the word fasting to describe a *starving* situation. Written possibly in ignorance, these books are grossly inaccurate and unfair to the reader, for they discourage fasting, especially the total fast. Even more reprehensible is the fact that many doctors still do not differentiate between fasting and starving.

When I explain the groundlessness of fears about *fasting,* I encounter the classic underlying inhibitions: "But won't I feel hungry and keep having hunger pangs?" "Won't I be faint and weak and have to stay in bed?"

My response to these concerns is based on tens of thousands of observed fasting experiences.

You will not be hungry. Any so-called hunger "pangs" are simply normal gastric contractions or stomach spasms. They represent the *sensation* of hunger rather than *true* hunger. Much of what we think of as hunger is really the desire for sensual nourishment and for pleasure and for warmth and for affection and for relief from boredom, frustration or loneliness.

To a very large extent, "hunger" is a conditioned reflex. ("If it's noon, I must be hungry and therefore I must eat.")

False appetite and stomach rumblings in the first few days are fleeting. They can be immediately quieted with a glass of water. (You should drink a minimum of two quarts of water every day of the fast.)

You will not feel weak or faint. In fact, you may discover new reservoirs of strength and vitality.

The very act of eating can be exhausting; it takes a lot of energy to digest food. When the body is freed from that chore, it naturally feels lighter and much more vibrant.

Not even during a lengthy fast should you stay in bed. As a matter of fact, the more activity, the better—within reason, of course. Exercise expedites the fasting process. It works as an appetite depressant by slowing the flow of insulin.

For decades the magazine *Physical Culture* reminded its readers that "fasting is an excellent agent for purifying the blood, and the majority of people who fast usually experience an increase in their ability to think more clearly. The five special senses of seeing, hearing, tasting, touching, and smelling become more acute during a fast."

As a psychiatrist, I am more than commonly aware of how attitude shapes the texture of any experience. What we expect in a situation is what we usually experience. If we approach something with an irrational dread, our unconscious may contrive to bring about adverse effects. As a colleague has wisely observed, you are practicing medicine on yourself every day as far as your own personal health is concerned.

There is simply no reason to be afraid of fasting.

Fasting is a revitalizing, reconstructive way of life which is healthful and inspirational. It is an adventure; it enriches body and soul. It is also, in the words of *Time* magazine, "the oldest, surest and quickest way to get rid of excess fat."

2.

Revitalization

Vogue magazine described fasting as "the newest and the most ancient practice. A religious rite. A historic mode of cleansing. A conditioner for meditation. A tool for consciousness-raising, for demonstration and protest."

Fasting can be defined in two words: *No eating.*

Purely speaking, it is the total abstention from caloric intake. It is a "diet" consisting only of water.

The definition of this discipline which surely is as old as man has become muddied in contemporary usage. One hears people say they're going on "a fruit juice fast" or "a vegetable juice fast" or "a bread-and-water fast." Some people say they're fasting when they eat a skimpy meal. A prominent California politician said he was "fasting by necessity—not choice" with a lunch of orange juice and a granola bar on the run. I have even read medical reports of fasts lasting 80 to 100 days—or longer. This is not possible! During a fast, appetite leaves on the fourth or fifth day. If the fast is not ended arbitrarily, appetite returns by the twenty-fifth to thirty-second day. When one continues to abstain from food after appetite returns, he is no longer fasting—he is starving!

The pure (water only) fast is a regimen which confers multiple benefits. To quote the second-century Greek physician Athenaeus, it "cures diseases, dries up bodily humors, puts demons to flight, gets rid of impure thoughts, makes the mind clearer and the heart purer, the body sanctified, and raises man to the throne of God." One of my colleagues has observed that fasting "hurriedly stops the intake of decomposition toxins. It gives the organism a chance to catch up with its work of excretion. It helps remove the toxins in the tissues. It causes the body to consume its excess of fat."

One of fasting's most alluring attractions—if not its *most* popular—is the dramatic loss of weight it accomplishes. It is "the ultimate diet" because weight is lost so much more quickly and easily than by any other weight-reduction method.

People who have a problem with weight basically have a problem with eating. Diets restricting the intake of certain foods or those top-heavy with other foods repeatedly fail because they do nothing to alter attitudes about food and eating. One can gain a new perspective on food and one's relationship to it by making fasting part of one's way of life—by fasting at regular intervals, preferably one day each week or three consecutive days in each month.

It is the somewhat overweight—but decidedly *not* obese—individual who feels most motivated to fast. He or she has gained weight and has enough self-esteem to want to look, feel, and actually *be* his or her best. (The "typical" faster is definitely not the compulsive overeater with deep-seated psychological disturbances. Such a person probably needs professional counseling and a thorough biochemical examination.)

Fasting improves personal appearance. The net result of weight loss is always a trimmer, more youthful appearance. The skin has a better color and texture after a fast. The eyes become clearer.

Fasting is a rejuvenating process; it can turn back the clock. Television's *Phyllis*—Cloris Leachman—likes to spread the word that fasting is a solution to the problems of the body. "It's simply wonderful. It can do practically anything. It is a miracle cure. It cured my asthma."

Miss Leachman thinks of all the water she drinks while fasting as "the fountain of youth." The minimum of at least two quarts a day serves a three-fold purpose:

(1) it prevents dehydration; (2) it stifles feelings of hunger; (3) it supplies minerals.

Drink the water even if you're not thirsty. Man can live a long time by water alone—but not by air alone.

Any kind of water whose chemical identification reads H_2O is fine. It should be at room temperature. I recommend bottled water, if it is available, rather than tap water. Most tap water contains chlorine and fluorides, manufactured chemicals. At a time when you are trying to cleanse your system, you should not be ingesting more chemicals. During a fast, many people find the taste and odor of tap water offensive.

I am sometimes asked if the water drinking doesn't add weight. It doesn't. When you eat nothing, the water you drink will be eliminated. The principal organ of elimination of water is not the kidneys but the skin with its millions of pores.

Alcoholic beverages must be avoided. Alcohol is highly caloric; during a fast, it can also be gravely injurious. This restriction can also serve as an obligatory start for anybody seriously wanting to resolve a drinking problem.

The longer the fast, the greater the chance the taste and yearning for alcohol will diminish. We have discovered that as the body and the palate purify themselves, they begin instinctively to reject the very *idea* of harmful substances.

It has been gratifying to see how many problem drinkers have been helped by a fast of even one week. Patients whom I would describe as heavy drinkers but not alcoholics routinely find their pattern of drinking modified. One prominent journalist told me her fast of only a week had helped her cut down from at least six drinks a day to two drinks—and often to none.

Fasting can also help break the self-destructive habit of smoking. I have had a number of patients who were able to give up smoking after a fast of only five or six days. None reported withdrawal symptoms or any desire to return to smoking. Fasting succeeded where all

the New Year's resolutions—and other efforts—to stop
smoking had failed.

The director of a weight-control camp in upstate
New York is a remarkable example of someone who
became an ex-smoker through fasting. She had smoked
for thirty-seven years before going on two four-day fasts
separated only by one day of light eating. She has not
touched a cigarette since.

One of my patients told me how *her* fast had succeeded in "curing" even her boyfriend's addiction. On
their first date after she had fasted and broken her
smoking habit, she backed off from his kisses. "My
God, the way your mouth smells!" she exclaimed. "I
can't kiss you. It would be like kissing an ashtray." It
was a variant of the old ultimatum "The lips that touch
liquor must never touch mine!" Happily, her boyfriend
made the right—and healthy—choice, deciding that
kisses are better than nicotine.

A spectacular anti-smoking success story is related
by Dr. Agatha Thrash of Yuchi Pines Health Institute in Seale, Alabama. She claims that 3,000 people—every participant in the program—have been
"cured" permanently of their smoking habit through a
five-day regimen. It begins with a day of total fasting,
then a day of modified fasting (juices). On the third
day, bread is added to the diet; on the fourth, vegetables; on the fifth, nuts. The regular diet is resumed on
the sixth day. Dr. Thrash, a Seventh-Day Adventist, is
convinced "a day or two of fasting—quickly clearing
the body of nicotine and other toxins—will do most
people more good than any amount of medical advice
or treatment."

Not all people who fast have made such a clean and
total break with a smoking habit, but most report they
are smoking less—and enjoying it less.

We now have evidence fasting can be an effective mo-
dality for breaking the drug habit. The tranquility of a
longer fast seems to obviate the need to return to artificial "highs" and escapes through "tripping."

Fasting can be a boon for insomniacs. Usually kept

awake by tension and anxiety, many find they are finally sleeping well. During a two-week fast, one of my correspondents reported, "I have been able to sleep through the night—every night—for the first time since I was a child." On the other hand, I have heard of fasters who find their energy level so elevated they cannot get to sleep. I advise anyone having trouble sleeping to exercise more than usual; exercise is a natural tranquilizer. A fast should replace tranquilizers, antidepressants, pep pills and barbiturates, anyway.

Reactions after a longer fast have included: ". . . tunes you in with the gentle voice of nature"; "I noticed a heightening of ethical and spiritual awareness. . ."; ". . . incredible euphoria"; and ". . . the occasion for a profound and insightful inner journey. . ."; it's like a month's vacation in the mountains or at the seashore."

3.
Getting Into It

You have decided to improve your life by fasting for a day or two or longer. You have rid your mind of all the false notions. You have your doctor's go-ahead. You are thoroughly familiar with the manifold benefits of the experience and you know millions of other people are doing it at this very moment.

But still you hesitate. You keep putting off "the day." You tell yourself you'll start tomorrow. Or next week.

How to translate good intentions into action? How to break through the procrastination?

There are ways of "psyching" yourself up.

If you are completely new to fasting, try skipping a meal or two on the day preceding the fast. This will give you a "taste" of discovering how easily you can get along without eating.

I tell all those fasting under my supervision that the first day or two may be trying but they will soon be quite comfortable.

First you must ignore the nay-sayers, who are always with us . . . the ones who are forever predicting something won't work or will have dire results. Negative feedback often comes from well-meaning friends and members of the family. Bear in mind you are doing something perfectly safe—something you chose to do, something that will benefit you, something *you can stop any time you wish.*

My colleague in Moscow, Dr. Yuri Nicolayev, who supervised tens of thousands of long fasts, told me his fasting unit had a two- to three-year waiting list because former patients enthusiastically extol the experience and results.

Fasting is popular because it is easy and because it works!

It is not possible to describe definitively the fasting experience, any more than one can describe the feeling of parachuting or hang-gliding. As Kafka put it, "Just try to explain to anyone the art of fasting! Anyone who has no feeling for it cannot be made to understand it." Reactions indeed vary over the entire spectrum of human response. An individual may feel different from one day to the next, but mostly he will feel good. "Even a one-day fast informs the body it can sacrifice food in good stride," noted Joan Gussow, chairman of the program in nutrition at Columbia University's Teachers College. "People are very flexible."

Two spa operators in England had notably effective ways for getting their guests "up" for the fast. Patients at Shrubland Hall Health Clinic were told to think of fasting as a rest, not a deprivation. Lady Julia de Saumarez of Shrubland said, "Rest should be encouraged in every part of the body—muscles, bones and the entire digestive system. When the patient realizes that fasting is in no way analogous to starving, his mental attitude is much more positive and rewarding."

Keki R. Sidhwa, who supervised about 5,000 fasts ranging from two days to as long as two months at his Shalimar, urged his guests to read up on fasting. Case histories serve to dissolve doubts and fears, and to convey the experience of fasting as a pleasure, not a punishment.

The Buchinger Kliniks in Germany and Spain have reminded their guests that fasting brings complete relaxation. They tell them to think of fasting as "an utopian vacation," and recommend at least a fortnight of doing without food.

Timing can be an important factor in "getting into it." A dentist in Connecticut who likes to fast 24 to 36 hours twice a week told me he had found it psychologically difficult to start fasting after a dinner and then not to eat again until breakfast two mornings later. He hit upon the easier regimen of starting the fast after breakfast and continuing through lunch the following day. When he gets up that second day, he tells himself he'll be eating again in just a few hours and energetically goes about his business.

One of my correspondents, a concerned citizen, finds the best way to get "in the mood" to skip meals is to remind herself of "disquieting" food facts reported on a NBC television program by Betty Furness, the consumer advocate: "More than 5,500 chemicals are put into our food supply, directly or indirectly, by the food processors [Miss Furness said] . . . the computerized plant, the chemical laboratory, is likely to be the basic source of our food . . . the fact of the matter is, the best scientific minds today are not able to tell us which food chemicals, if any, will cause us bodily harm, when they will strike, and how many of us will be hurt . . . We know there is strong evidence that some of the damage may not show up for years."

It all comes down to convincing yourself it is good for you to fast—which it is!—and get on with it.

Most people do the short fast alone. It's simply something they've chosen to do for a day or two or three, and they manage very well even when others around them are eating and drinking.

Understandably, it is easier for some people to fast by making it a companionable venture, especially if it's for an extended period. You don't have to go away to a spa to have company. Persuade a member of the family or a good friend or a fellow worker to fast with you. This way you can swap progress reports. You'll have a booster to cheer you on. You can check out each other at the scales or before a full-length mirror to see who's losing more weight, who's getting trimmer.

(Maybe someday you'll be able to avail yourself of the new M.I.T. electronic scale. It is so sensitive that the most minuscule fluctuation in weight is registered.

You could stand on such a scale and *see* yourself losing weight from one minute to the next.)

Having a goal can help. If the swimming pool season is only a week away, images of how the "new" you will look in a bathing suit can be a powerful incentive to "shape up" the quickest way. An impending prom or a wedding or a trip to Europe or any other occasion when you'd want to look your best can provide the motivation for launching your fast.

Here is another suggestion that works with many of my patients. Figure out how much time you will save by not eating. My co-author Eugene Boe found preparing for a business trip eats up so much time that he fasted the two or three days prior to departure in order to save about four hours each day.

Think of all the money you also save by not eating.

There are exciting ways to spend the saved time and money.

Why not reward yourself for being so good? One ingenious device is to pay yourself for each pound you lose. The reward money could easily come out of the money you save on food bills with every day you fast. By fasting just one day a week, you save nearly 15 percent of your weekly food bill.

The financial incentive also seems to work very well in research projects. At the Veterans Administration Hospital in Salt Lake City, subjects in an experiment were paid to fast. The men reportedly threw themselves into the project with great fervor.

Another novel approach for getting "set" comes from a friend who has fasted many times. She suggests using my refeeding schedule *in reverse*. That is, if she plans to fast for three days, she allots herself three days of "training." She begins with my Day Three postfast menu (see page 29) and day by day reduces rations (see pages 28-27) until the fourth day—the first day of a three-day fast. A three-day fast preceded by the three-day "refeeding" program leads to an impressive weight loss and, I might add, a trimmer figure.

Generally, the initial experience with fasting breeds the desire to do it again. And again and again.

Bernarr Macfadden, an indefatigable exponent of fasting, once remarked, "A weekly fast is necessary to insure the continuous possession of the vigor and vitality we all crave. Intoxicating health is indeed life's greatest treasure and any effort made to acquire it pays rich dividends." Mr. Macfadden was still parachute-jumping at the age of 83.

The best "psyching up" stratagem has to be the simple reminder to yourself that fasting is good for you. It produces results at a pace and of a quality not obtainable with any of the diets that come along every season and are widely tried and found wanting.

There are 27,960 different methods for losing weight on file in Washington. Most of them have a brief vogue and are abandoned. Fasting has outlived them all.

4.

Business As Usual

For me a day of fasting is like any other day. I go about my usual busy routine, seeing patients and making my hospital rounds. The only difference is that I don't eat. By not eating I find I have extra time to catch up on my reading and writing. I also have increased stores of energy. (I was not surprised to read that a group of young men in a University of Minnesota experiment *improved* their performance at *hard* work with *periodic* fasts.)

Every healthy person who fasts for a day or two or for many days should be able to go about normal social and work routines—"business as usual."

There is no psychological or physiological reason for cutting back on activity. Fasting for short periods is perfectly compatible with a full work load and an active participation in play. You will instinctively know if you have to cut back a bit.

The very definition of fasting would seem to supply the answer to the question, How does one fast?

The answer is simple: *Stop eating.*

That's it. You don't eat. Nothing could be simpler. Your diet consists of water—and lots of it! At least two quarts a day.

A caution about fasting at home: do not tempt or test yourself needlessly.

Put the thought of food out of your mind. Skip the food pages in newspapers or magazines. Don't riffle through cookbooks and menu files. Walk briskly by restaurants without pausing to examine menus posted in

windows. Bypass supermarkets and bakeries and delica-
tessens and ice cream parlors.

If you are a homemaker, you cannot possibly escape all encounters with food. You will probably have
to go on preparing meals for the rest of the family.
This presents a challenge, but not an insuperable one. I
know a mistress of the house who even hosts lovely
dinner parties while fasting. In many households where
the homemaker is fasting, another family member takes
over the chores of shopping and cooking.

Lorraine Orr, owner-moderator of the syndicated
radio program (over 400 stations) called "Good Living," tells me she is able when she fasts to put in several
extra hours in the office while her husband takes over in
the kitchen. If the Orrs are having guests, he serves her
during the cocktail hour a Perrier "highball" that looks
for all the world like the vodka and soda she normally
has. During a fast, Mrs. Orr finds it "a pleasant surprise" that she has high energy even at the end of a
long dinner party.

A 29-year-old free-lance writer and children's magazine editor, Denise Van Lear, fasted several times
during a heavy writing project. She was greatly helped
by an imaginative friend who surprised her with a
"grande bouffe." He set the dining table with the usual
cutlery and napery and brought on large pitchers,
crystal goblets, soup bowls, and cups—all filled to the
brim with water. He then touched a match to tall, per-
fumed candles. "At that moment I loved him more
than ever," she later told me. She had such renewed
gusts of energy that she took to scrubbing and cleaning
her whole house from stem to stern; she had a compulsion to make it as "immaculate" as the fast was making
her. She would bound out of bed at six o'clock in the
morning ready to tackle anything.

Since he began fasting on a regular basis, the director
of the television department of a busy talent agency
said he has never performed better in his work. "I have
so much energy, I always feel great. I am a very happy
man," he told me. "I've got everyone here fasting now."

On a trip to the West Coast, I read in the *Los Angeles Times* of a construction engineer who enjoyed a ten-day fast while his fellow workers and family all continued to eat ravenously. He socialized with "the boys" at lunch over a glass of water on the rocks. At the dinner table he savored the same for his "entree," while the rest of the family packed away "tons of food." After dinner he jogged his usual two miles. The *Times* reported he lost the desired amount of weight "with no effort at all."

Barbara Pinsof, A.S.I.D., who heads her own interior design firm in Glencoe, Illinois, got up each morning of a five-day fast with "more bounce and energy than customary." She astounded herself with her ease at fasting. "I turned off the hunger response totally," she said, "and felt very well. Never hungry, I turned out a tremendous amount of work that week—and lost 12 pounds in the bargain."

A woman interviewed by *W,* the Fairchild weekly which reports on high fashion and the antics of "society," reported: "I don't lead a quiet life while fasting; I just continue being as busy as usual. I fast when I have something important coming up, or when I'm bored, or to clean out my system. Fasting gets me quite excited. It must be nervous energy."

A newspaper woman in the South gets "tons and tons" of things done while fasting. During a single "lunch" hour she ran errands that had been accumulating for weeks. (She also became aware of the hordes on the street who "are always stuffing their face with cold drinks, potato chips, candy, and peanuts—in public yet.") In San Francisco, an entertainment response analyst, Sebastian Stone, uses his extra hours to meditate, to get in touch with his system, nerves, and tensions.

Feelings of fasting-induced euphoria or light-headedness can distort perception. This raises the important question of whether to drive a car during a fast. There are differences of opinion on the subject. I know of a man in Denver who deliberately fasts during a three- or four-day automobile trip so that he won't have to pull into "greasy spoons" along the way. And I know of a spa where the guests are permitted to take day-long motor trips in the historic surrounding countryside.

I see no objection to driving during a short fast if the person is in average good health and is not fasting to alleviate an illness. Performance at the wheel should be keener with the increased alertness.

The body usually adapts itself easily to the fasting experience. Most people breeze through even an extended fast without experiencing discomfort, since the process of nutrition continues as though food were still being consumed. Some fasters report fleeting headache or nausea or faintness or dizziness or palpitations as the body rids itself of waste.

Many working people I know fast in the pursuit of self-improvement. They use their meal hours and meal money to attend adult education courses, redecorate their apartment, or take tennis or language or music lessons. Some go to a popular movie over the lunch hour, when queues aren't as long as after work.

Single people who are accustomed to cooking for themselves appreciate fasting as a way of escaping from the boredom and nuisance of shopping, cooking, and cleaning up for one.

5.

How to Lose Weight Without
Eating—*and Keep It Off*

We are spending billions annually to lose weight.
But despite the peer—and medical—pressures to shed
our excess weight, we are heavier today than we were
15 years ago.

And the incidence of obesity is still increasing, according to Columbia University's Institute of Human
Nutrition. Women are gaining weight at a faster rate
than men, particularly women in the 30–40 age range:
40 percent of all women in this group are now classified
as obese.

Thirty-five percent of *all* Americans (including children) are overweight and 20 percent are obese. (Obesity—which is defined as being 20 percent over one's
preferred weight—is our number one health problem.)
The obese person has a 40 percent greater likelihood of
dying from heart-related diseases than a person of a
preferred weight. Anyone 25 pounds overweight is in
effect carrying around a 25-pound bag everywhere he
goes.

America has imprisoned itself in a tunnel of fat. This
has been true from the beginning of the republic. Benjamin Franklin, who knew whence he spoke, noted, "I
saw few die of hunger, but of eating? 100,000!" Too
many mouths still act as litter baskets and garbage
dumps.

The change in our diet in recent times is reflected in
these grim statistics: between 1929 and 1958, per
capita consumption of fresh fruits and vegetables de-
clined 30 percent while consumption of processed foods
increased 152 percent.

The nation badly needs to go on a diet. It should do something drastic about excessive, unattractive, life-threatening fat. It should get rid of it in the quickest way possible—by fasting.

How much weight can you lose on a fast?

A great deal. More than you could on any kind of diet.

The rate at which you lose weight is generally in proportion to the degree you are overweight. You can lose up to 5 pounds on a one-day fast, up to 10 pounds on a weekend fast, and from 12 to 20 pounds or more on a week-long fast. Men, because they tend to be larger and heavier, lose weight more quickly than women.

Given the mathematical equation of weight loss— we must burn up 3,500 more calories than we consume in order to lose one pound—you might well ask how is it conceivable to lose so much weight so rapidly. The explanation is simple. Our body is about 70 percent water. Eating causes the retention of fluid. When we stop eating, large amounts of water are eliminated from the body. The scale is pound-blind: it treats a pound of water the way it treats a pound of fat. Each weighs exactly the same.

During the "first fine careless rapture" of a fast, pounds drop off rapidly. Understandably, progress is not quite as impressive thereafter.

In the beginning the body loses accumulated water. This accounts for the considerable weight loss. Then it begins to "burn" its fat, a much slower process. After a week or more, the rate of weight loss decreases to about a pound a day. The body is now getting its nutrients from its well-stocked pantry of "preserves." This "pantry" is ample to supply all nutrition needs for several weeks—and sometimes longer for the obese —without drawing on any of its emergency rations.

Too many people in their desperation to rid themselves instantly of extra pounds choose methods that are as dangerous as being overweight itself. Chief among these methods are the "anti-appetite" pills, which are gulped down indiscriminately, and restrictive diets that allow only one type of food. How much better—and how much more effective—it is to take the health-promoting approach of a fast!

The late Director of the Federal Bureau of Investigation, J. Edgar Hoover, was known to abhor flab on his agents. In a thinly disguised novel about the F.B.I. called *Don't Embarrass the Bureau,* agents of the bureau are instructed to fast in advance of a visit from The Director. One of the officers tells his men, "I expect to be looking at some pretty lean bodies around here within the next few weeks. There's absolutely no reason why we should be criticized for something like excess weight. I've been told a person can lose as much as 20 pounds in one week if need be."

Andrew Unger has written in *Moneysworth,* "Compared to a standard program like that of Weight Watchers or Dr. Atkins, fasting is the superior form of weight control. A typical fast is for the goal of losing 12 to 15 pounds. Think of it as losing a Don Carter bowling ball."

The insurance companies have been telling us we might live a lot longer if we weighed considerably less than even the recommended weights on most charts. The insurance companies, as we all know, are geared to the profit motive. I should think it would make good business sense for them to underwrite fasting treatments for obese people rather than pay out policy money for premature death caused by such obesity-related complications as high blood pressure, diabetes, or elevated cholesterol levels.

Every day's mail brings cheering accounts from correspondents who have overcome their weight problems through fasting. Here is a sampling of "case histories":

> I was able to lose 22 pounds within eight days. On two subsequent fasts I lost another 25 pounds. My wife has also lost weight faster by fasting than by any other means. Fasting for short periods of time is certainly the fastest and most predictable method I

know. . . .—Dr. M. N. N., Perth Amboy, New Jersey.

I was severely overweight, about 100 pounds or so. I was able to take off all 100 pounds. . . . (Why is it that we lavish so much money on the maintenance of our automobiles to keep them from conking out and so little concern on keeping our bodies from conking out?)—A. G. G., Manhattan, Kansas.

In two weeks I lost 27 pounds and all my funny little aches and pains disappeared.—G. F., Taunton, Massachusetts.

I was feeling sluggish, sleepy and overweight, and ready to retire from my insurance business when I went on my first fast. After seven days I had lost 23 pounds and was able to return to my office and work a full 14-hour day as I hadn't done for years. I now fast at least a day a week. . . .—S. G. R., Oxnard, California.

On my most recent birthday, which coincided with Oxfam's Fast Day, I determined I must lose excess weight and take stock of myself. I decided to fast, and now have lost over 20 pounds. I did yoga exercises at the same time—mainly upside down ones for circulation: headstands, shoulder stands, and "the plow."—Ms. S. R. C., Iowa City, Iowa.

As a nurse I should have known better. But I let myself go all the way up to 245 pounds. I went on a four-day fast and lost 15 pounds. To be continued. . . .—Ms. B. A., Trenton, New Jersey.

One of the most satisfying rewards of being the author of *Fasting: The Ultimate Diet* was to learn that the regimen set down in the book had inspired weight-reduction programs on a company-wide basis. At Intermatic, Inc., an electrical products manufacturing concern in Spring Grove, Illinois, a "Diet Derby" was instituted. Each entrant was to be paid three dollars for each pound lost, providing at least 15 pounds were lost in a year. The company made no recommendation on how to lose weight. Each employee was allowed to pursue her or his own method; there seemed to be as many methods as there were reducers. Some ate only candy bars. Others consumed only salad dressings. A few tried yoga. And there were those who believed more things are wrought by prayer than this world dreams of.

About halfway through the program, Intermatic's president, Jim Miller, noted that the participants were disappointed with their progress. Not many pounds were being shed, or kept off. At this point he distributed a copy of *Fasting: The Ultimate Diet* to each person still in the program. Here is what he told me:

> The reactions to your book were very favorable. As one person and then another tried fasting and reported that the desire for food diminished greatly after the first day, others were encouraged to try it, too. When I gave the awards at the end of the program, most of the men and women with whom I talked attributed their successes to "the ultimate diet." There was agreement that fasting is much easier than dieting, and that fasting gives immediate results.
>
> There was no doubt, from my observation, that those who had succeeded in fasting had a sense of accomplishment and a much improved outlook. They reported having a sense of "renewal." There is a psychological impact as a result of fasting beyond merely loss of weight.

The 137 employees in the Intermatic Derby collectively "lost" more than half a ton. In addition, there was the auxiliary benefit of the appreciable drop in blood-pressure levels which always accompany a fast.

As a result of the Diet Derby and the national attention it attracted, Mr. Miller is "convinced a major segment of our population has a great desire to be thin. It seems to me a very large number of young people in particular are carrying excessive weight and they feel somehow it is unfair. We live in a permissive society where the child can get away from his parents, his teachers, and even his church—only Mother Nature seems to demand self-discipline."

I agree with the Intermatic president when he says that far more important than the money the "losers" won are the *years* they've won—the years added to their lives. Overweight can be *very* dangerous. Anyone who rids himself of excess weight is a much healthier and more effective person.

Once you resume eating, some weight gain *naturally* occurs. The body retains fluid, which translates into weight because of the sodium content in food. For a time after any fast this will be more weight than is metabolically balanced for the amount of calories being consumed.

The best way to keep your weight down after the initial fast and to keep reaching new low levels is to make fasting a way of life.

If you fast principally to lose weight, the ultimate goal should be to keep off the pounds you lose. Fast on a regular basis: one day every week, or every weekend, or three days every month, or even one-week to ten-day periods twice a year.

Between fasts, try to keep caloric consumption in alignment with caloric needs. Such a program should lead to successive lower readings on the scale.

A return to a previously unhealthy life-style can take away the blessings gained through fasting. This is a fact I cannot over-emphasize.

6.

After-the-Fast Menus

When you start to eat again, you must not burden the digestive system—now cleansed and rested—with too much food or the wrong kind of food.

When you have fasted for even a few days, your system will require less food than you had been accustomed to eating. (You will not have accumulated hunger or appetite.)

After a longer fast—of a week or more—the body is enlightened. It puts appetite into alignment with the body's *real* needs for energy. The probability is you will now consume only as much food as your body burns.

In the words of a veteran faster, "A fast heightens awareness of the individual's integral relationship to the nourishment that feeds the body."

Gorging food after the fast or trying to compensate for "lost meals" could have lamentable consequences. At the very least you would surely regain weight you had shed. You could also become ill.

The wise person eases into a sensible refeeding program. Easy does it if you want to continue feeling wonderful and to keep your weight at or near its new low level.

In effect, the body is re-educated by a fast. It "unlearns" habits of overeating and "polluting." It is "born again." It inclines toward a natural state. It wants only as much food as is required for maintenance. It prefers the kinds of food that are natural to the taste and harmonious to the digestive system.

My new after-the-fast eating schedule is an agreeable

and palatable alternative to the refeeding program that appeared in *Fasting: The Ultimate Diet*. The menu plans are intended to keep your weight at—or below —its post-fasting level. They are also designed to provide a healthy, nutritious, high-energy interlude between the completion of the fast and the resumption of regular meals. They are balanced and complete in all the essential nutrients.

Throughout the after-the-fast diet you may drink as much water as you wish. *You should drink at least one quart of water every day.*

It is advisable to eat slowly and to chew carefully. (Good advice anytime.)

You should not add salt to your food.

You should adhere to the refeeding schedule for the same number of days you fasted. If you fasted five days, for example, you should follow the schedule through Day Five.

Most people who fast of course continue their normal work routine. It is suggested they prepare their refeeding meals on arising in the morning. Meals to be eaten during the day can be put into thermal containers and taken along to the job.

When you return to a regular eating pattern, the likelihood is that you will be eating more selectively and austerely, which is all to the good.

The Day One Menu

The day's menu consists of one pint of boiled water mixed with one pint of grape juice or orange juice or apricot juice.

Sip two or three teaspoons of the mixture every ten to fifteen minutes throughout the day, finishing the full quart by bedtime.

The Day Two Menu

The menu consists of undiluted grape juice or orange juice or apricot juice.

Drink half a cup (four ounces) of the juice on arising and an additional half a cup every two hours until bedtime. You will drink one quart of the fruit juice if you are up 14 hours today.

The Day Three Menu

The menu of five meals consists of one quart of yogurt and one pound of apples.

Wash and grate the apples, and mix with the yogurt.

Divide the combination into five equal meals.

Eat a meal every three hours, preferably at 9:00 A.M., noon, 3:00 P.M., 6:00 P.M., and 9:00 P.M.

The Day Four Menu

The menu of five meals consists of one quart of yogurt, one pound of apples, and one-half pound of carrots.

Wash and grate the apples and carrots, and mix with the yogurt.

Divide the combination into five equal meals.

Eat a meal every three hours, preferably at 9:00 A.M., noon, 3:00 P.M., 6:00 P.M., and 9:00 P.M.

The Day Five Menu

The menu of five meals consists of one and one-quarter cups of yogurt, one-quarter pound of apples, one-quarter pound of carrots, one teaspoon of honey, a vegetable salad (described below), and two walnuts.

Wash and grate the apples and carrots, mix with the yogurt, and add the teaspoon of honey and the walnuts. Divide the combination into five equal meals. Eat at the same hours as on Days Three and Four: 9:00 A.M., noon, 3:00 P.M., 6:00 P.M., and 9:00 P.M.

At the noon meal, have also a vegetable salad consisting of one boiled potato, one cup of raw fresh chopped cabbage, and one chopped onion—dressed with one tablespoon of vegetable oil.

The Day Six Menu

The menu of four meals consists of one and one-quarter cups of yogurt, one-quarter pound of apples, one-third pound of carrots, two teaspoons of honey, two walnuts, one-third pound of farmer cheese, and a vegetable salad (described below).

Wash and grate the apples and carrots, mix with the yogurt, and add the honey and the walnuts. Divide the combination into four equal meals. Eat a meal every four hours, preferably at 9:00 A.M., 1:00 P.M., 5:00 P.M., and 9:00 P.M.

At the morning meal, add the farmer cheese.

At the 1:00 P.M. meal, add a vegetable salad consisting of one boiled potato, one cup of raw fresh chopped cabbage, and one chopped onion—dressed with one tablespoon of vegetable oil.

The Day Seven Menu

The menu of four meals consists of one and one-quarter cups of yogurt, one-quarter pound of apples, one-third pound of carrots, two teaspoons of honey, two walnuts, two-thirds pound of farmer cheese, a vegetable salad, and a cup of oatmeal or buckwheat topped with milk.

Wash and grate the apples and carrots, mix with the yogurt, and add the honey and the walnuts. Divide the combination into four equal meals. Follow the same meal schedule as for Day Six: 9:00 A.M., 1:00 P.M., 5:00 P.M., and 9:00 P.M.

At each meal have one-fourth of the farmer cheese.

At the morning meal, have the oatmeal or buckwheat topped with milk.

At the 1:00 P.M. meal, have the vegetable salad consisting of the same ingredients as that for Day Five or Six.

The Day Eight Menu

The same menu and schedule of four meals as Day Seven.

The Day Nine Menu

The same menu and schedule of four meals as Day Seven, except for the addition of one tablespoon of sour cream mixed with the day's portion of farmer cheese.

The Day Ten Menu

The same menu and schedule of four meals as Day Nine, plus a cup of vegetable soup at the 1:00 P.M. meal.

The Day Eleven Menu

The same menu and schedule of four meals as Day Ten.

The Day Twelve Menu

The same menu and schedule of four meals as Day Eleven, with the addition of three teaspoons of vegetable oil and a pint of orange, grape, or apricot juice.

At the morning, 1:00 P.M., and 5:00 P.M. meals, have a teaspoon of vegetable oil. (You may wish to add the vegetable oil to your vegetable salad.)

At each meal have one four-ounce serving of the fruit juice.

The Day Thirteen Menu and Beyond

Continue the menu and schedule of four meals of Day Twelve for as many additional days as are necessary—that is, if you fasted for fifteen days, you should adhere to the Day Twelve diet for three additional days.

My after-the-fast schedule is one of several in popular use. Two estimable alternative refeeding programs were kindly supplied for presentation in this book by Joy and Robert Gross, who operated the Pawling Health Manor in Hyde Park, New York. The programs are appropriate for the seven-day refeeding period after a week-long fast. Amounts may be adjusted to individual desire. (I do not use either of these programs for breaking the fast.)

First day after the fast
4 ounces fresh orange juice mixed with 4 ounces water. Sip slowly, every three hours.

OR:

Breakfast:	1 grapefruit
Lunch:	6 ounces clear vegetable broth
Dinner:	1 grapefruit

Second day after the fast

Breakfast:	8 ounces fresh orange juice
Lunch:	1 small piece watermelon
Dinner:	2 oranges

OR

Breakfast:	8 ounces fresh tomato and celery juice
Lunch:	1 pound fresh grapes
Dinner:	8–10 ounces vegetable broth

Third day after the fast

Breakfast:	8 ounces fresh carrot and celery juice
Lunch:	1 or 2 ripe tomatoes, couple of stalks celery, 3 ounces pot cheese
Dinner:	Medium-sized vegetable salad, baked potato

OR:
Breakfast: 1 grapefruit
Lunch: Several slices ripe fresh pineapple, 8–10 strawberries
Dinner: Green salad, steamed baby peas, 3 ounces pot cheese

Fourth day after the fast
Breakfast: 8–10 ounces fresh grapefruit juice, 3 ounces sunflower seeds
Lunch: 1 ripe banana, 1 ripe pear, ½ cup raisins
Dinner: 8 ounces carrot and celery juice, medium-sized green salad, baked potato, steamed asparagus

OR:
Breakfast: 1 grapefruit, 1 orange
Lunch: 1 large ripe tomato, 4 ounces alfalfa sprouts, 2 stalks celery, steamed whole green beans
Dinner: Medium-sized salad, medium portion steamed brown or wild rice, steamed zucchini squash

Fifth day after the fast
Breakfast: 1 medium-sized piece watermelon
Lunch: 8 ounces vegetable soup, 3 or 4 ounces cottage cheese, several leaves romaine lettuce
Dinner: Medium-sized green salad, 1 ripe tomato, 3 or 4 ounces sprouts, ½ avocado

OR:
Breakfast: 8 ounces carrot and celery juice, 3 ounces pine nuts
Lunch: 3 or 4 large nectarines
Dinner: Medium-sized green salad, baked potato, steamed broccoli

Sixth day after the fast

Breakfast: Fresh strawberries, 3 ounces raw cashew butter

Lunch: 1 or 2 ripe mangoes, 8 ounces fresh ripe blueberries

Dinner: Large green salad, steamed lima beans, ½ avocado

OR:

Breakfast: 1 or 2 grapefruits

Lunch: 2 ripe bananas, 3 ounces natural dates, 1 pear

Dinner: Large green salad, steamed eggplant with tomatoes, 3 or 4 ounces pot cheese

Seventh day after the fast

Breakfast: Ripe papaya (as much as desired)

Lunch: Fresh blueberries, 1 or 2 ripe peaches, 3 ounces ricotta cheese

Dinner: Finger salad—romaine lettuce leaves, celery, carrot sticks, green pepper slices, endive; steamed yellow squash, steamed kasha

OR:

Breakfast: 5 or 6 soaked jumbo prunes

Lunch: 6 or 8 ounces fresh vegetable soup, fresh celery sticks, 3 ounces imported Swiss cheese

Dinner: Large green salad, vegetable casserole— alternating layers of ripe tomatoes, eggplant, green peppers, potato, parsley, in baking dish. (Soybean oil may be used in bottom of pan and if liquid is needed, celery juice may be used.)

7.

After the After-the-Fast Menus

You have shed many pounds during your fast and approached or arrived at approximately your ideal weight.

From my experience, there is no doubt you will have a much better chance for permanent weight control after fasting than after any diet. The system now *wants* to reject food in excess of the needs of the body.

You should now be able to gain a new perspective on food and a new relationship to food that can keep you from overeating or from eating undesirable foods. Fasting and a sensible refeeding program have led to this desideratum.

The after the after-the-fast diet should consist of modest amounts of all fruits and vegetables currently available. It should favor fresh fruits and vegetables, whole grains and cereals, nuts and seeds, poultry and fish. It should be sparing of meat, sweets, and fats, and free of any food containing sugar, and it should be low in salt.

There are many healthful diets providing "three squares" a day that still allow for weight control. Here is one basic menu I recommend—and basically follow:

Breakfast: Half a grapefruit or an orange or the juice of either. A cooked or a granola-type cereal plus one tablespoon of unprocessed bran five mornings a week, one egg the other two mornings. One butterless piece of whole wheat or rye toast with honey. A cup of café au lait consisting of one-third cup of coffee and two-thirds cup of boiled milk, or herbal tea with lemon.

Lunch: A cup of plain yogurt with nuts and figs or raisins two or three days each week. Fruit or a vegetable salad on the other days.

Dinner: Fish or fowl. A huge bowl of salad with lots of vegetables. A baked potato. For dessert, a piece of cheese and an apple or a pear.

For a great many people, fasting leads to a vegetarian life. Most fasting retreats serve only vegetarian meals after the refeeding program. They urge their guests to adopt new dietary habits, all-vegetarian if possible, on returning home. Some prepare menu plans for the departing guests.

Without departing from the conviction that diet, where possible, should be individually tailored, Shrubland Hall Health Clinic in England made available to patients on departure a general diet sheet. (I do not use this sheet.) The advice it gives is this:

On Waking:
Hot or cold water with lemon and honey. *This is essential.*

Breakfast:
N.B. This is the most important meal of the day. On no account leave it out.

Either one-half grapefruit or one orange or apple.
Select one:

1. Boiled egg, one crispbread with a little butter (one-half ounce total daily allowance).

2. Four ounces plain yogurt with wheat germ or bran and honey (one ounce total daily allowance).

3. One-half cup Muesli *well soaked* in boiling water *or* fruit juice, *not* milk.

4. Prunes (soaked in hot water for 24 hours). All-bran *or* plain bran for extra bowel movement should be added if required.

5. Two lean rashers grilled bacon and one tomato.
(The above may be alternated.)
One cup China or herbal tea or coffee (not instant) *or* small glass *fresh* fruit juice. No milk (one-half cup

allowed daily *if absolutely necessary*). No sugar (noncaloric sweetener if essential).

Mid-morning:
  Nothing if possible. Otherwise choose one:
  1. Small glass fresh fruit or vegetable juice.
  2. Cup of tea or coffee. No milk or sugar.
  3. One cup marmite or soup. One low-calorie fruit or vegetable, e.g., apple, carrot, celery, *if you need it.*

Luncheon:
  First course (if desired)
  Select one: consommé, tomato juice, grapefruit, melon.
  Main Course
  Mixed salad containing as many different raw vegetables as possible. Select six from: lettuce, watercress, fennel, grated raw cabbage, grated white cabbage, grated carrot, grated raw beetroot, chicory, endive, onion, cucumber, raw mushroom, shredded raw spinach, mustard and cress, celery, radish, green pepper, grated celeriac.
  One teaspoon cider vinegar *or* lemon juice for dressing if desired.
  Select one from: boiled egg (total weekly allowance of four), six prawns or shrimp, two ounces grated cheese *or* milled nuts, four ounces cottage cheese, small baked potato (may be included twice weekly), avocado pear.
  Third Course
  Two crispbread or one slice wholemeal brown bread. Very little butter. Tea *or* coffee (see breakfast).
  Do not have cheese, fruit, or eggs twice in the same meal.

Tea Time:
  One or two cups China or herbal tea (with lemon if desired).
  One teaspoon honey or brown sugar is beneficial at this time of day and may be taken in addition to the daily allowance.
  No coffee, no milk, nothing to eat.

Dinner:

First Course

None if taken at luncheon; otherwise select from luncheon choices.

Main Course

Select two vegetables from: carrots, parsnips, celery, onions, leeks, French beans, Brussels sprouts, cauliflower, spinach, broccoli, tomatoes, marrow squash, cabbage, green peppers, eggplant, sea kale, mushrooms, courgettes. (These must be boiled or steamed, grilled where applicable, never fried.)

Salt may be used in cooking but very little added afterwards.

Select one medium portion from: two ounces grilled liver, three ounces lamb chop, three ounces veal, three ounces roast chicken, two ounces lamb, three ounces turkey, four ounces steamed or grilled whitefish such as cod, sole, plaice, fresh haddock. No sauces. No gravy. (Cheese or egg dishes are suitable alternatives.)

Third Course (if required)

Select one fresh fruit from: peach, apple, melon, plums, apricots, pear, cherries, pineapple, black or red currants, blackberries, orange, gooseberries.

Beverage

One or two glasses of dry wine with dinner, if absolutely necessary for social or business reasons.

Otherwise, for the purpose of this diet, regard all alcoholic beverages as unsuitable and avoid them.

Do not have the bedtime drink if you have had wine.

You may reverse the suggested luncheon and dinner.

Bedtime:

Optional drink. Hot water flavored with honey and cider vinegar or lemon. Herbal tea, vecon, or marmite. (Avoid stimulants such as coffee and China or India tea on retiring. You do not need a milky drink.)

Unsuitable foods:

White bread, white sugar, cakes, pastries, puddings, biscuits, white rice, spaghetti, pastas in general, thick soups, sauces, gravies, olive oil, dressings, milk, milk shakes, fat meat such as pork, sausage, beefsteak, fat fish such as pilchards, herrings, sardines, breakfast cereals (except Muesli), jams, marmalade, syrup, canned foods, dried foods, sandwiches, snacks, chocolate, sweets, ice cream, cream, dried fruits such as dates, figs, sultanas, prunes, apricots, rhubarb, bananas. (Peas, potatoes, brown sugar, honey, ham, bacon, butter, margarine only in amounts indicated in the diet.)

The Shrubland diet, the dietician told the guest, was carefully balanced to meet all nutritional requisites for good health and a sense of well-being. You were strongly advised to adhere to it and not to tamper with it in any way. It was designed to give maximum variety and generous freedom of choice according to individual taste. Therefore, you should find it socially acceptable and personally satisfying to your appetite; your family, social, and business requirements can be met without preventing you from following the diet strictly. Easy preparation and food prices have also been taken into careful consideration.

Again, the above diet and advice came from Shrubland; they are not mine.

8.
The Adequacy of Vegetarian Diets

Today, there is increasing interest in vegetarianism. The reasons are various. First, there is the continuing problem of inflation, which is bringing higher and higher costs of food in general and meat in particular. Also, there is a growing sensitivity to the hunger and food shortages confronting most of the world's population. And there is the increasing suspicion there might be a link between some illnesses and a diet heavy on meats.

The person who fasts frequently comes to prefer the vegetarian regimen.

This reorientation raises the question, can vegetarian diets satisfy nutritional needs?

The word *vegetarian* is *not*—as one might presume —derived from the word *vegetable,* but from the Latin *vegettus,* which means "whole, sound, fresh, lively."

All vegetarian diets exclude meat, poultry, and fish. But vegetarian diets differ significantly in what they do contain.

The four most common variations of vegetarianism are:

1. A pure or strict "vegan" diet. It excludes all foods of meat-poultry-fish *origin* (eggs, milk, cheese, ice cream, yogurt, etc.).

2. The ovo-lacto vegetarian diet. It allows eggs and dairy products.

3. A lacto vegetarian diet. It permits dairy products but excludes eggs.

4. A fruitarian diet. It is restricted to raw and dried fruits, nuts, honey, and olive oil.

Large populations of the world have subsisted on

diets that are essentially, if not literally, vegetarian. According to the Scriptures, the human diet was to consist of fruits, seeds, and nuts. Later, herbs and vegetables were "approved." The Creator said, "Behold, I have given you every herb-bearing seed that is upon the face of all the Earth and every tree in which is the fruit of a tree-yielding seed, to you it shall be for meat."

The latest official statistic—it goes back to a Gallup poll taken in 1943—indicated that in the United States alone there were 3-million vegetarians. The present concern for ecology and a contented, harmonious life —combined with new nutritional knowledge—has boosted that total, I would guess, to at least 12-million.

Despite the fact man has survived perfectly well throughout history on fleshless food, there is periodically raised the concern as to the amount and proper kind of protein that vegetarian diets provide.

The quantity and the quality of protein are a concern in *any* diet. The quality of protein is determined by the kinds of amino acids—the building blocks of protein—the food contains. Eight of the 23 constituent amino acids in protein are considered vitally important to the diet. They are referred to as "essential." They are available in plant sources. Killing of animals for protein is indeed an arrogant exploitation of Earth's finite resources.

Soybeans and chick peas are rich in high-grade protein. So are lentils, nuts, and seeds. Bread, cereal, vegetables, and fruits are not quite as rich. Combining these foods with as much variety as possible provides a diet adequate in protein, and in all other nutrients as well.

Effective protein combinations—which complement each other to make whole or complete proteins—are beans and rice, cereal and milk, and macaroni or other pastas and cheese.

On a vegetarian diet, one must consume larger quantities of food to get adequate nutrients. This does not mean loading up excessively on any foods on the approved list. The recommended wide variety of foods in vegetarian diets is necessary to insure adequate intake of the more-difficult-to-obtain vitamins (folic acid and vitamin B_{12}) and minerals such as calcium and iron.

(For impoverished populations having no choice *but* to be vegetarian, there is the promise of a new type of corn as an answer to protein needs. An international team of scientists has developed a species designated as Opaque-2. It contains large amounts of lysine, which is lacking in ordinary strains of corn. Opaque-2 has about doubled the effective protein content of normal corn, surpassing the amount found even in milk. Sanat K. Majumder, associate professor in the Department of Biological Sciences at Smith College, tells us that under proper agronomic conditions more than 200-million people who live in the tropical corn regions can derive dietary benefit, both quantitatively and qualitatively, from these strains.)

In vegetarian diets, two daily servings of high-protein alternates—peas or beans, nuts, peanut butter, vegetable "steaks," dairy products or eggs—are recommended. If dairy products are not used, calcium and riboflavin can be obtained in adequate amounts by liberal intakes of dark green leafy vegetables and fortified soy milk.

While most of the 4,000,000,000 people on Earth may not be getting enough protein, many affluent Americans are probably consuming too much. Nutritionists once advised that the daily diet should contain one gram for every two pounds of weight. This seems to be in excess of what our body actually requires. The government now says that adults require about 48 grams of protein per day. This figure may be on the high side. Controlled experiments have shown the average person can function perfectly well with protein intakes of only 30 to 35 grams per day. (By the way, even steak rates as "junk food" when it contributes to an excess of protein consumption, in light of the definition that "junk food" is anything the body does not need.)

However many grams of protein we are taking in, we may be much better off if the protein is not from animal sources. Studies by Dr. John W. Berg and others at the National Cancer Institute link colon cancer with high consumption of beef. A study of Seventh-Day Adventist men—most of whom are strict vegetarians—found they have about 75 percent *less* than the expected rate of intestinal and rectal cancer and less than half the expected rate of all types of cancer.

Another study concluded that in populations habitually subsisting on a diet *high* in animal foodstuffs —including dairy products—heart disease was far more prevalent than in vegetarian populations.

Dr. George L. Blackburn, assistant professor of surgery, Harvard Medical School, has gone on record as saying that a vegetarian diet incorporating egg and milk sources of protein "is more than adequate to maintain proper nutrition and resulting health."

Dr. Glenn D. Toppenberg, of New England Memorial Hospital, Stoneham, Massachusetts, goes so far as to claim from personal experience that children can flourish on vegetarian diets. Writing in *The New England Journal of Medicine,* he discusses vegetarian child-raising at first hand: "My three children are now the third generation of my family to have never tasted meat, and it certainly has not been detrimental to our health. My 13-year-old high school boy—6′3″ and size-14 shoes —can hardly be accused of retarded physical growth, and all three children are at the top of their classes at school and are socially well adjusted."

Lancet, the British medical journal, supports Dr. Toppenberg's view: ". . . many field trips have shown protein provided by suitable mixtures of vegetable origin enable children to grow as well as children provided with milk and other animal protein."

Corroborating studies involving 112 vegetarian and 88 nonvegetarian adults, adolescents, and pregnant women were reported in the *Journal of Clinical Nutrition* as follows:

1. The average intake of nutrients of *all* groups exceeded those recommended by the National Research Council, with the exception of adolescent "pure" vegetarians.

2. Nonvegetarian adolescents consume more protein, but there is no evidence that an ovo-lacto vegetarian diet failed to provide adequate diet for them or for expectant mothers.

3. There were no significant differences in height, weight, and blood pressures among the groups, but the "pure" vegetarians weighed an average of 20 pounds less.

4. Cholesterol was higher in the nonvegetarian groups. The "pure" vegetarian diet, whatever its shortcomings, is *cholesterol-free*.

Studies conducted by Dr. Frederick Stare of Harvard and Dr. Mervyn G. Hardinge, now dean of Loma Linda (California) School of Health, confirm that vegetarians have consistently lower levels of serum cholesterol than do meat eaters. Meat eaters may also be bothered by poor elimination; food with low fiber content, such as meat, moves sluggishly through the digestive tract.

Many large institutions, such as Smith College, have begun to de-emphasize meat in its meals. At Hampshire College, the director of food services says "food is a subject that students take seriously." At prestigious Stuyvesant High School in New York City, yogurt is now offered in the cafeteria.

Some of our high-circulation periodicals that depend on advertising revenues from meat packers are even endorsing the vegetarian regimen. "The staunchest meat-eaters have come to accept the fact that you don't have to eat red meat, poultry, or fish to get the kind of protein your body needs and can use," according to a *Redbook* article. The magazine published menus for meatless meals providing "balanced" protein. Among the entrees were Brazilian black beans and rice with salsa, two-cheese rice balls, sukiyaki with noodles, linguini with walnut sauce, French bean pot, lentil potato soup, Chinese slivered eggs and mushrooms, cheese-and-potato pie, and sweet and pungent chick peas.

The *Reader's Digest* reprinted an article from *Today's Health* attesting that protein from non-flesh foods can be an adequate nutritional substitute for meat protein. It was observed that "vegetarians are thinner, in better health, with lower blood cholesterol, than their flesh-eating fellow ctitizens."

A *Ladies Home Journal* feature asserted that the heartiest appetites could be satisfied healthfully with ample protein without dependence on meat. The *Journal* published recipes for "main" dishes such as nutty bean loaf, fried stuffed zucchini, Mexican chili baked with soufflé topping, spinach Parmesan pie, and ratatouille crepe stack.

McCall's presented in tabular form "the price of protein," establishing that all the plant-food sources cost but a fraction of meat protein, and concluding that "cutting down on meat wouldn't be a hardship; it can be an exercise in ingenuity to get maximum protein for minimum cost."

Accelerating interest in vegetarianism is a natural consequence of our health-endangered industrial society. Many people—of all ages, not only the Woodstock generation—are seeking alternative life-styles of "purer" foods requiring neither the destruction of animals nor the use of chemical fertilizers and pesticides. They seek a mode of eating that enhances spiritual values and bio-ethics. A 19-year-old woman from Orangevale, California, summed it up in *Seventeen* magazine: "Vegetarianism is a more economical, healthful and ecologically sound way to eat."

9.

The Strenuous Life

Contestants with the training and stamina to participate in long-distance running competitions are typically lean. It is amazing how deceiving appearances can be. These stripped-down, almost cadaverous looking bodies actually have enough reserves to sustain *tremendous* exertion.

Many outstanding runners who are in tip-top condition program fasting into their schedules as faithfully as they do road-work.

Pennsylvanian Park Barner goes without food before long-distance runs. Within a two-week period he ran 36 miles and a double marathon (52½ miles).

A Swede, Erik Ostybe, abstains for several days before a marathon.

Germany's Meinrad Nagele, once severely overweight, credits a series of fasts with helping him "shape up" at the age of 46 and become a winner in the World Veterans games.

Murray Rose, of England, was a gold medal winner in the 1956 and 1960 Olympics. (He was a vegetarian; he had never eaten meat.)

Another English devotee of fasting, Ian Jackson, declared, "I feel better when fasting than when eating. I feel more alert, lighter on my feet, more collected, and calmer than usual." For the *Runner's Diet,* Jackson lyrically recalled what it was like after a week of fasting: ". . . my body was moving effortlessly, gliding along with no urgency. Everything was smooth, mellow and peaceful. My senses were incredibly heightened, finely tuned in. I felt a natural unity with the dark trees and the drifting mist. The sighing of the wind in the pines, the clear bird calls and the occasional creaking of branches seemed to penetrate gently into the very center of my being. With a combination of elation and gratitude, I let my body move on while my mind and my senses touched their home . . . pure awareness of joyful existence."

Dick Gregory, who is in his mid-forties, participated in the Boston Marathon while fasting. As a personal bicentennial celebration, he ran from Los Angeles to New York—a total of 2,980 miles; an average of 50 each day—without taking any solid food.

Nineteen Swedish men, who ranged in ages from 18 to 53, and worked mostly at sedentary jobs, hiked from Kalmar to Stockholm, a distance of more than 300 miles. They ate no food during the 10 days, averaged 30 miles a day, and were in "the best of spirits" on reaching the capital, having taken the whole thing in stride.

Fasting has had its adherents in boxing. To get under the 126-pound maximum weight for the division, featherweight Johnny Chacon fasted for a week to lose 16 pounds. A heavyweight contender, Harry Wills, "the Brown Panther," would fast for a month each Spring in order to lose at least 40 pounds and get into fighting trim.

A famous University of Chicago professor of physiology, Anton Carlson, discovered the endurance and energy of a football team rose markedly after a three- or four-day fast.

It may come as revolutionary news to television viewers of sports and food commercials that *many* professional athletes are foregoing food before competition. The American College of Sports Medicine, based in Madison, Wisconsin, has promulgated the opinion that the traditional pre-game meal is not essential. "In fact, we have observed over many years that some of the truly great athletes ate absolutely nothing before competition."

The hearty pre-game meal is a long-cherished old wives' tale handed down from coach to coach without discernment of its potential harm. Before an event, the traditional thinking went, athletes had to stock up on marbled steaks, mounds of scrambled eggs, gallons of milk, and racks of toast and honey. It is now understood by many coaches the energy needed to digest such a meal is deflected from performance. The food acts as an extra load, contributes to fatigue, and lodges in the stomach long after the event is over.

Ernst van Aaken, a medical doctor who coaches runners, believes frequent fasts lead to greater endurance. "It is necessary," he observes, "to have fasted frequently for at least 24-hour periods in order to perform with a completely empty stomach. Frequent fasts build up carbohydrates in the liver from reserves already present in the organism." He believes endurance activities can be carried on for days with almost no food.

But need I point out athletes (in common with the rest of us) should eat sound, balanced meals containing protein, carbohydrates, and the other essential nutrients when not being called upon for an expenditure of extraordinary amounts of energy. And logically, it seems to be best to eat nothing at all the day *of* and the day *before* the competition. The body does not depend on food consumed just *before* or *during* heightened activity. It performs with the reserves it has accumulated over a period of time. Talk it over with your team doctor or trainer.

During a fast, blood sugar stays on an even keel within the normal range. Those who *eat* experience a rise in blood sugar, which brings on an outpouring of insulin and a lowering of the blood sugar level. For the athlete there may be the accompanying conditioned craving for a Hershey bar or a Gatorade "break."

An article in *Nutrition Reviews* also challenged the notion that athletes should pack away a feast before going into action. At the same time it questioned the wisdom of carbohydrate-loading athletes in training, pointing out that its effectiveness is doubtful. As a matter of fact, the fasting process releases ketones into the bloodstream, blunting hunger and providing a source of energy for metabolism.

(We are of course talking throughout this chapter about mature, fully developed athletes—not growing grade school or high school youngsters. *Young people during their growth period should never fast except in a medically controlled situation.*)

With the whole world now sports wild, it is time we discard many myths concerning the care and feeding of athletes. In reading a provocative book entitled *Food for Fitness,* I found myself in solid agreement again and again with its iconoclastic views. The book, by the way, was published by World Books, a California publishing enterprise specializing in books and manuals on active and intense sports: cross-country skiing, swimming, bicycling, running, gymnastics, the martial arts, canoeing, hiking, and rafting.

"Nowhere is superstition more flagrantly and unquestionably adhered to than in diets," declares *Food for Fitness.* It then proceeds to slaughter many a sacred cow:

"Every body needs milk." Absolutely not so. In fact, there are many people, including a large segment of the white population and an even greater percentage of the black population, who cannot digest it.

"Every body needs bread." Again not so. And again there are those who literally cannot stomach it. Their systems are unable to produce enzymes necessary to break down starch and protein simultaneously.

"Steak for breakfast is best on game day." Steak at that time is a drag, not a lift. Its protein doesn't convert into energy quickly enough to be helpful. It also overburdens the elimination system at a time when it is already overworked with heavy perspiring.

"Candy bars give you a boost." They do—for a matter of moments—and then drop you like a runaway

express elevator. "The entire 'quick energy' myth is a giant rip-off invented by the very industry that led you to eat things that make you feel sluggish in the first place."

"Protein gives you a quick lift before an event." In the energy derby, protein comes in last. Of all nutrients, it takes the most time to digest. Fruit sugars, starchy foods, and fats give a quicker "pick-me-up." (*Seventeen* magazine has said, "The traditional steak dinner or pre-game breakfast to turn players into dynamos is nothing but a high-priced myth.")

Even the American Dietetic Association dismisses the notion of high-protein intake as a *sine qua non* for athletes. "Protein utilization does not increase during exercise when fat and carbohydrate contribute sufficient energy," the A.D.A. maintains. "Diets high in protein and protein supplements have been advocated for athletes on the premise that body muscle is protein and an ingestion of an excess of protein would stimulate muscle growth to improve strength."

(*The Physician and Sportsmedicine* magazine reports studies in animals and humans have not demonstrated any benefits from eating excessive amounts of protein. "In fact, one of the most impressive developments in clinical nutrition has been the treatment of chronic renal disease by *lowering* protein intake." The periodical asks, "If such good results are possible by restricting the intake of protein, is excessive protein intake healthy for normal human beings? Is there perhaps even danger in over-consumption of protein?")

"Drinking anything is bad before, during, or after strenuous exercise." Nonsense! Athletes have been known to die of dehydration. Body temperature soars during dehydration, bringing on the threat of a fatal heat stroke. In less than an hour, athletes can sweat away dangerous amounts of fluid. They can suffer dizziness, nausea, and a dangerously elevated pulse rate if they don't replenish themselves constantly. Don't worry about bloating. Drink up. (But no beer. One beer can lower your heat tolerance for as long as three

days.) Any thirst should be slaked immediately—and preferably with plain unadulterated water.

The biggest myth of all, as has been amply demonstrated, is that anybody engaging in strenuous exercise must—in order to turn in a peak performance—stoke up before participating. It is also probable that the athlete who eats more with the intent of becoming stronger and playing better only becomes fatter, develops excessive eating habits, and stimulates fat cells to multiply and enlarge.

To paraphrase an old maxim: He travels fastest who travels lightest.

What about "the strenuous life" during a fast for the non-athlete and the person not in peak physical condition?

As you might imagine, I cannot agree with the contention, voiced especially by fasting spa operators, that fasting should be a time of complete physical rest even for the healthy person. I have discovered no reason why the healthy person who is fasting for a few days shouldn't continue with the type of exercise to which he or she is *accustomed. Failure to exercise, in fact, brings on fatigue.* Exercise slows down the activity of the pancreas and this prevents a lowering of the sugar level and avoids fatigue.

Dr. Otto Buchinger, who directed tens of thousands of fasts, observed that "we do not conserve any energy by mollycoddling our powers. It simply is not true that exercise impedes rather than enhances weight loss during a fast or that one loses more weight by resting than by being active. Instead of losing fat, the immobile body mainly loses valuable muscle and organic albumen."

But do only as much as you can comfortably do. Avoid doing anything to the point of exhaustion, of course—always good counsel.

If you don't usually exercise, the fasting period would be a good time to get into the habit of walking. You can accomplish a lot of walking during hours otherwise spent preparing food and eating. I insist those people who fast under my supervision walk briskly for at least one hour every day of a short fast and at least three hours every day of a long fast. I break the fast of anyone who can't or won't.

10.

The Contemplative Life

*All fasting is . . . a yearning of the soul to merge in
the divine essence.*

—Mahatma Gandhi

In the quest for serenity and wisdom and heightened
states of awareness, fasting has been a revered discipline. Its origins go back millennia, to the Eastern mys-
tics and to the prophets of the Old Testament. It was
popular with the savants of ancient Greece and Rome
and of the Renaissance. "If practiced with the right in-
tention, it makes man a friend of God," said Tertullian,
the Roman theologian. "The demons are aware of that."

To gain mental and spiritual rewards, the membership
of the Self-Realization Fellowship* fasts in accordance
with the teachings of its guru-founder, Paramahansa
Yogananda. In his "bible," *Man's Eternal Quest,* the
rewards of fasting are delineated:

    1. The spirit within becomes disassociated from the
demands of the body as the body itself is freed from
gross habits.
    2. Fasting gives rest to the overworked organs, the
bodily engines.
    3. Fasting gives rest to the life force itself, reliev-
ing it of extra work. The life force is the sustainer of
the body, and through fasting it becomes self-sup-
porting and independent.
    4. Overeating every day of the year creates many
kinds of disease.

---

*The Fellowship was founded in the United States nearly six decades
ago to create understanding among the religions of East and West.

5. Undeviating regularity in eating, whether the system needs food or not, is a curse to the body. The more you concentrate on the palate, the more disease you will have. To enjoy food is fine, but to be a slave of it is the bane of life.

6. The physical effects of fasting are remarkable. A fast of three days on orange juice* will repair the body temporarily, but a long fast will completely overhaul it. (Persons in good health should experience no difficulty in fasting for three days; longer fasts should be undertaken only under experienced supervision. Anyone suffering from a chronic ailment or an organic defect should fast only upon the advice of a physician experienced in fasting procedures.) Your body will feel as strong as steel. But if you want a permanent overhaul you must at all times watch what and how much food you take into your body. There is a great metaphysical science behind fasting. Jesus reminded us of this truth when He said, "Man shall not live by bread alone. . . ." Two things keep you bound to Earth: breath and bread. In sleep, however, you are peacefully unaware of the need for either breath or food; your spirit is detached from body consciousness. Fasting uplifts the mind in the same way.

7. Fasting lets the mind depend on its own power. The mind tells itself: "The solids on which the body used to depend are nothing more than gross condensations of energy. You are pure energy. And you are pure consciousness."

8. The mind, in learning to depend on itself through fasting, can do anything: conquer disease, create prosperity, or realize the supreme goal of life—finding God.

Tennessee Williams, in his autobiography, *Memoirs*, recalls being stranded as a young man in a remote desert area of California. He had neither food nor money to buy food. After the third day of his involuntary fast, he observed "with considerable astonishment" that he no longer felt hungry. "The stomach contracts, the gastric spasms subside and God or some-

---

*I believe juice with all its calories and tea or soda or coffee should *not* be consumed during a fast. A water-only diet is the true fast and is what I recommend for purest results.—A.C.

body drops in on you invisibly and painlessly injects you with sedation so that you find yourself drifting into a curiously and absolutely inexplicably peaceful condition, and this condition is ideal for meditation on things past and passing and to come, in just that sequence."

11.

The More Beautiful People

Before appearing on a television series to discuss "the ultimate diet," Hugh Downs told me he fasts every Monday to control his weight. He got the idea while visiting Lion Country Safari in California. He learned lions in captivity are not fed one day a week because of their conditioning; in the wilds they had been used to going without food occasionally. "While I do not consider myself a lion, gustatory or literary," Mr. Downs remarked, "I share a mammalian evolution with the species and it occurred to me that I, too, might be healthier if I suspended bombarding my stomach with viands one day a week. The dial of my metabolism appears to be set in such a way that I run about eight pounds heavier than I prefer when I eat as comfortably as I like to eat; the alternative is that I can maintain the weight I desire by running slightly hungry always."

By fasting on Mondays, Mr. Downs finds he can eat pretty much what he wants the other six days and maintain desired weight. His appetite is less on the three days following a one-day fast—still another example that fasting regulates or moderates appetite. "Fasting is indeed *not* starving," he observes. "But unfortunately, as I have traveled through various parts of the world for television productions, I have met people who *are* starving. Maybe if we can get better distribution methods and more people doing themselves good by fasting occasionally, the planet will be a pleasanter place."

George Romney, former Presidential candidate, Michigan governor, and president and board chairman of American Motors, fasted at least one period a month. "It is a means of building spiritual strength, and is at the same time good for the body. The funds saved are contributed to my church for use in assisting those in need. Fasting," he adds, "strengthens control over our appetites, thus contributing to self-mastery."

California Governor Edmund ("Jerry") Brown, Jr. was 15 pounds overweight when he embarked on a series of fasts. He would fast for 24 hours or 48 hours or sometimes longer. "The fasting idea was spreading around the Governor's office," said Trish Cruskie, a nutritionist in the California Health Department, "the same way it seems to have spread to many other circles in California."

Vidal Sassoon, the internationally renowned hair stylist, has fasted for a 36-hour period every month. He was described by fashion arbiter Eugenia Sheppard as looking 20 years younger than his acknowledged 48.) What harm can there be, he asks sensibly, in skipping four of the 90 meals we usually eat in the course of a month? He says that the monthly fast makes him feel "marvelous, very light, very pure," while giving his liver and digestive system "a great rest. I've found that it brings me great clarity of thinking and stimulates me to all sorts of new ideas for my work." Mr. Sassoon discovered fasting nearly a score of years ago when he was in a state of nervous exhaustion. His friend Kenneth Haigh, the actor, suggested he pack a sweat suit and a copy of Camus' *The Stranger* and hie himself to a health farm for a week of fasting and rest. In his best seller, *A Year of Beauty and Health,* Mr. Sassoon extols the virtues of fasting as the first step in a long-range program to improve health and appearance. "Remember, you are not depriving your body of food. You are rewarding it with rest. Fasting is a way of reaching full potential."

Helen and Scott Nearing were in their mid-seventies and mid-nineties, respectively, and still fasted every Sunday. Mrs. Nearing explained that it was "to give the body and the housekeeper (me) an occasional rest and vacation." The Nearings, who pioneered the back-to-the-land movement in the 1930s—hacking out "the good life," first in Vermont and now in Maine—had not seen a doctor in four decades. "If we were to become ill," Mrs. Nearing told me, "we would fast for an extended period."

John Hill, who founded the public relations firm of Hill and Knowlton half a century ago (it is now the largest public relations firm in the world), first fasted as a young man of 21. He describes that first fast of three or four days as being "exceedingly salutary." In middle age he fasted for seven days after a long siege of knee trouble, which, he said, no doctor or specialist had successfully been able to diagnose or treat. The disorder disappeared and never returned. Mr. Hill, still active at 86, fasted on an intermittent basis and found it "a beneficial practice."

Gwen Davis, the novelist and screenwriter, met some "spectacularly healthy people" while she was visiting Liza Minnelli during the filming of *Lucky Lady* in Guaymas, Mexico. Those denizens of good health told her that fasting was "a wonderful trip" for their body. "As I had spent most of my life trying to give a wonderful trip to my brain," she wrote me, "I thought it was time to give an equal chance to my slightly 'too, too solid flesh.' " At the end of a two-week fast, she said she never looked or felt better. "My skin, my hair, my body tones were all improved. I actually seemed taller." She now fasts every Monday and tries to fast a second day during the week if she does not have obligatory business lunches or dinners every day. "I always feel better when fasting. The big trick for me is not to think about food. At times this is difficult—bean sprouts and crisp bell peppers and sunflower seeds seem sinfully good." Whenever she finishes a major writing project, Ms. Davis likes to go to the desert and fast for five days "to rid myself of the anxiety and tension that has accumulated." When she loses the struggle to keep from smoking, she fasts to cleanse her system of nicotine and to cut down on the habit. "Fasting never interferes with my normal work routine," she says. "When I did a two-week fast in Guaymas, I completed a first draft of *The Aristocrats,* a novel about a movie company on location. I fasted off and on while writing a book of meditations called *How to Survive in Suburbia When Your Heart's in the Himalayas.* It wouldn't surprise me if fasting contributed to the clarity of thought I needed for the meditations."

Douglas Auchincloss, the socialite, told a Fairchild publication he was casual about fasting, preferring to fit it into his schedule so that it did not interfere with social engagements. He found Sunday "the good day." He lost about two and one-half pounds on a one-day fast. "I find fasting makes me feel better afterwards. It's no hardship at all."

Dr. John C. Lilly, famous for talking to dolphins and whales, reduced his weight from 210 to 143 pounds on his first fast, 38 years ago. At the first sign of gaining weight, he goes on brief, "corrective" fasts. "It is encouraging," he said, "to see this new generation doing its own myth-making in the areas of fasting and food."

12.

The Medical Orthodoxy

If fasting is so wondrous, the question might well be asked, Why aren't more of us in the medical profession championing it?

I am afraid an attitude has developed among some of us that it is impolitic and risky to try new knowledge or any procedure that did not bear the stamp of approval of our colleagues in the profession, especially if it happened to be a controversial procedure. Though fasting has been around for five millennia, it is controversial still.

The observation has been made that "the human brain is not only an organ of thinking but an organ of survival . . . it is made in such a way as to make us accept as truth that which is only advantage." The advantages of closing one's mind to some fundamentally new truth preclude release not only from the burden of learning something new but also from *unlearning* that which is familiar and therefore secure and comfortable.

The primary discoveries of Harvey, Lister, Pasteur, Ehrlich, and many others were vigorously resisted from within the profession. René Laënnec was expelled from his medical society after inventing "the stethoscope"—a sheet of paper rolled into a tube; one end was placed on the patient's chest and the other was applied to the doctor's ear. Some members of the American Medical Association still contest the need for vitamin supplements (as witness the roaring controversy raised by Nobel Prize-winner Linus Pauling's book *Vitamin C and the Common Cold*), minerals, and X-rays.

I find it incongruous that doctors inexperienced in the fast immediately talk about fasting in terms of danger, yet casually prescribe enormous doses of tranquilizers and sleeping pills for periods of many years, as well as antibiotics and other drugs having the potential for unpleasant, sometimes irreversible side effects, addiction, and a high incidence of morbidity. The attitude of aloofness on the part of the medical profession has allowed fasting to drift almost exclusively into the hands of non-medical groups.

Recently, the Associated Press reported that "the diet of affluent Americans able to afford any foods they choose is less nutritious than it was [in the 1960s]. The problem: We are overfed but remain undernourished. As a result, experts say, 10 percent of the population may be anemic and 35 percent overweight."

There is a popular cliché about weight control: "The only way to lose weight and keep the weight off is to have three balanced, nutritious meals a day." But this approach is simply too frustrating for many people who have a weight problem and need the psychological boost of achieving a quick initial weight loss to motivate them to continue the weight-loss program. It also betrays a lack of flexibility and imagination in exploring alternate methods to the regular eating regimen for solving weight problems. The obese "relish" fasting because it is so quick, helpful, and easy; my reluctant colleagues should seriously consider this fact!

There *is* progress to report. Research into fasting is under way at many medical centers, here and abroad. Members of the Academy of Preventive Medicine have begun to fast patients. *The Journal of the American Medical Association* published the opinion that fasting provides the best method of self-discipline needed by the obese—"one that can be repeated with beneficial effect." *The New England Journal of Medicine* has published the view that fasting is "a valid experience for any otherwise healthy person who has failed to relieve the weight problem by every other method."

What interested me most about the prolonged protest fast of Gary Gilmore, the Utah prisoner demanding execution, was the reaction of his doctors. When Gilmore was two weeks into the fast and had lost 25 pounds, the doctors attending him said he could continue the fast for another month without difficulty. The prisoner obviously was in the hands of enlightened medical men.

13.

Fasting for Bodily Ills

In my earlier book on fasting, I put major emphasis on weight-reducing benefits. Overweight is the surpassing health problem in the nation, and I felt certain most readers would primarily be interested in learning about the easiest and quickest way to lose unwanted pounds. I therefore restricted myself in *Fasting: The Ultimate Diet* to several paragraphs about fasting for other health gains.

If I can believe the evidence of my eyes and ears, more people are fasting today than I would have guessed, and many of them are fasting therapeutically to stay well and to rid themselves of dis-ease.

Chronic diseases claim a crippling grip on 35-million of us. Fasting does *not* cure chronic diseases or anything else, but it has helped the body to heal itself of more distresses than we may dream.

In the sixteenth century, the illustrious physician Paracelsus called fasting "the greatest remedy." In Sweden thousands of members of the health organization Hälsofrämjandet fast for up to two weeks as a *preventive* measure. Their goal: "The total regeneration and rejuvenation of all functions of the body."

All of us who fast patients have files bulging with testimonials claiming relief from a whole alphabet of complaints ranging from asthma to viruses. Spa literature abounds with case histories of people who are said to have overcome the agonies of psoriasis, acne, peptic ulcers, constipation, hay fever, arthritis, colitis, varicose veins, dermatological diseases, anemia, eye diseases such as iritis and retinitis, rheumatism, gallstones, stress and nervous exhaustion, diseases of the digestive and respiratory organs—and yes, even the common cold.

A woman in Connecticut who is the secretary-treasurer of a factory in Bridgeport fasts to overcome bouts of arthritis. Each year she fasts for two periods, of ten days and five days, having learned, she says, "the subtle but clear language" of her body. Besides getting relief from her arthritis, she finds her skin after the fast "looks opalescent, clean, and clear, and my mind is sharp, my energy levels are tremendous. My body looks beautiful, I truly love myself, and I am once more happy with the entire world."

A Florida executive told me how fasting relieved his prostate problem. "In the 12th day of the fast my urine stream was free and broad for the first time in eight years. On the 21st day I had the first complete emptying of my bladder (no retention) in eight years."

Two colleagues report encouraging results with diabetics. But I cannot be too emphatic in warning that *no diabetic* should undertake a fast except under the closest medical supervision.

I have found a fast of four days to be an effective first step in detecting the origin of food allergies. With the body rid of all reactions from food, a series of direct testings with different foods is initiated to discover which contain the allergens. By introducing only one food at a meal, we can isolate the offending food or foods. Determining food allergies through fasting frequently gives better results than can be achieved by skin-testing.

In the winter of 1976 I vacationed in Mexico and visited Villa Vegetarina in Cuernavaca. The villa called itself "Mexico's rejuvenation resort." Besides fasting its guests, the villa offered a regimen of natural organic foods, sunshine, rest, yoga, and exercise. The villa's director, David Stry, spoke of healing rather than curing: "Only a ham can be cured." He found fasting allowed the body to strengthen its forces against many ills.

At the villa I met guests who assured me their maladies, aches, and disorders were being "healed." Before going there, some had given up hope of feeling well. Years of "doctoring," drugs, and surgery had proved ineffectual. Relief from advanced stages of arthritis seemed to be a recurring wonder at the villa. Mrs. O. W., for example, told me she had cortisone injections back home—to no avail—but after three weeks of fasting, followed by a vegetarian diet, she could walk up stairs again, lift her arms, and go to sleep—all free of pain. A 42-year-old asthmatic alternated fasting with small vegetarian meals, and told Mr. Stry that his miseries had finally vanished. A retired commercial airline pilot's serious varicose vein condition all but disappeared after a seven-day fast.

From other hygienic centers come similar reports of dramatic relief from arthritis and asthma after all other forms of treatment had failed.

From Shalimar, a health spa on the Eastern coast of England, Keki R. Sidhwa—its enthusiastic director who fasted patients for a quarter of a century—wrote me that most of his guests arrive suffering from "acute and chronic diseases of various kinds." He claimed the recovery rate through his fasting program is "85 to 90 percent."

More than 2,300 years ago, Hippocrates, "the father of medicine," made this observation: "Everyone has a doctor in him. We just have to help him in his work."

Otto H. F. Buchinger, who supervised tens of thousands of fasts, observed, "Fasting is . . . a royal road to healing for anyone who agrees to take it for the recovery and regeneration of the body."

Permit me once again to emphasize that a therapeutic fast must be under *strict* medical supervision. The fasting procedure is definitely not for everyone (see chapter 15), and individual testimonials mentioned must not be taken as unqualified approval for all who might fast. Every person is adaptable to fasting in a different manner and degree!

14.
Fasting for Mental Ills

Its realization was a long time coming, but the cliché "we are what we eat" is now understood to be as applicable to the state of our mental health as it is to our physical health. The quality of our nutrition indeed affects our behavior, our mood level, and even our sanity.

The necessity of good nutrition for maintenance of physical health was underscored by those who pioneered in the discovery of the vitamin-deficiency diseases and their cures early in the present century. It took another four decades, or until about 1945, for an understanding to develop of the relationship of nutrition to mental health. Around 1945, Dr. Yuri Nicolayev of the Moscow Psychiatric Institute was introducing the revolutionary concept that mental illness, particularly schizophrenia, could be helped through the recuperative powers of fasting and a revised diet.

Dr. Nicolayev, who fasted more than 10,000 mentally ill patients, reported unusually encouraging results with those patients who had failed to improve on all other treatment programs. Once given up for "hopeless," 65 percent of patients who experienced fasting therapy went on to achieve sufficient improvement to live and function outside of the hospital.

At least two out of every hundred persons on our planet suffer from schizophrenia in some degree. As my good friend Dr. Humphry Osmond points out, this dreadful disease knows no national or cultural boundaries and responds to no quarantine or immunization.

We have learned that with the increasing use of drugs in the treatment of mental and emotional disturbances there has been a corresponding increase in the number of patients who become drug-resistant. Other patients may have toxic reactions or develop other complications, some of which may be irreversible. For patients who do not respond to drug treatments, or who respond negatively, fasting is proving to be a valuable alternative.

In 1970 and again in 1972, Dr. Nicolayev invited me to observe in his therapeutic fasting unit and to discuss with him and his large staff my work in orthomolecular treatment. The Moscow Psychiatric Institute consisted of a 3,000-bed research center with a staff of 500 physicians. The fasting treatment was conducted in an 88-bed unit.

The fast itself lasted about a month. It was terminated when appetite returned, breath was fresh, the tongue became clear, and symptoms were alleviated—signs that a fast of any length should be broken.

After breaking the fast, the patient stayed in the hospital an additional number of days equal to the length of the fast. Refeeding began with a salt-free diet of fruit, vegetables, and some form of acidulated milk. The quantities of food were gradually increased. Meat, eggs, and fish were excluded. Bread was not offered until the sixth or seventh day.

About half of Dr. Nicolayev's patients who were examined after a period of six years had maintained their improved condition. Relapses occurred among those patients who added protein foods from animal sources to the prescribed diet. The maximum effects of the treatment were manifested two or three months after treatment was completed provided the diet had been followed precisely.

One form of schizophrenia prevalent in the U.S.S.R. and whose prognosis had *always* been quite poor responds positively to the fasting treatment. This syndrome is dysmorphobia. It is characterized by delusions of physical shortcomings, and the patient is obsessed by a fear of the escape of offending gases and odors from the body. He or she is convinced that everyone near can hear the sounds and smell the odors. There are usually accompanying convictions of being ugly and undersized and universally repellent. It is impressive that fasting can eradicate even paranoid delusions.

Other types of schizophrenia are alleviated during the fasting and recovery periods. The manic phase of manic-depressive illness can be brought under control in the first week of a fast.

My own experience with treating schizophrenics with fasting was conducted in Gracie Square Hospital in New York City. I made it a prerequisite for admission to the treatment that the subject had been ill with schizophrenia for at least five years and unresponsive to all prior forms of treatment. Another requirement was the consent of the patient and his family. Since the fasting treatment requires the patient's full cooperation, there is no hope of success unless the patient is acutely aware of the gravity of his illness and is willing to give more than passive consent to trying a different approach. I also stipulated that my patients stay out of bed and remain active. They could leave the hospital in the morning and take long walks about the city. (They were free to leave therapy whenever they wished.) They were required to walk, preferably briskly, a minimum of three hours a day. Paradoxically, without three hours of exercise daily, feelings of weakness developed and the fast had to be arbitrarily broken. If a patient willfully broke the fast by eating, treatment was stopped and the patient was discharged from the hospital.

Everyone drank a minimum of two quarts of water every day. If a patient failed—or refused—to drink this amount, I terminated the fast. Daily cleansing enemas and showers or baths were imperative. During the shower or bath, the patient was encouraged to stimulate circulation by using a loofa straw mitt for a washcloth. Patients who had been on medication were able to dispense with it by the end of the first week. Everyone in the program was required to give up smoking—and did.

The fasting period was tolerated surprisingly easily by these very ill people. There were some complications during the recovery period. These occurred mostly from overeating when protein was introduced into the diet. Patients soon learned they had to stick to the prescribed diet in the specified amounts. They had to stop eating before they felt full. In some, the protein addition to the diet produced a period of excitation, tension, or sleeplessness. Sleep medication was prescribed for these patients.

Of the 35 men and women who participated in my fasting project, 24 have not relapsed into illness.

These conclusions can be drawn about treating schizophrenic patients with the controlled fast:

1. While the fast of 25 or more days may lead to some degree of exhaustion, it also serves as a powerful stimulus to subsequent recuperation.

2. Fasting insures rest of the digestive tract, which in itself is a normalizing aid.

3. The acidosis induced by fasting probably plays an important role in neutralizing some of the toxins that may have contributed to the schizophrenic condition.

Schizophrenics have a higher protein level than non-schizophrenic people. Fasting therapy mobilizes the proteins in the body. The process peaks in about seven days. After the fast, the protein level is within normal range. Within three to six months the level tends to rise to the pre-fast level; it is another reason for undergoing recurrent periodic short fasts.

After the publication of *Fasting: The Ultimate Diet,* I heard from the former patient cited as an example of one who had been functioning effectively since completing treatment. He wrote me protesting my use of the word *effectively.* Apparently I had understated his case. "I am very successful in almost everything and happy," he wrote me, "and I think I can appreciate life far more than most people."

Dr. Abe Hoffer, of Saskatoon, Saskatchewan, who has written extensively on mental illness, still wonders why physicians—especially psychiatrists—"are so surprised when they hear of the beneficial effects of a fast. Many become as enraged over the fast as they are when someone mentions megavitamins. I have now seen severe and chronic schizophrenics who had not responded to any previous treatment—including megavitamins, drugs and electro-convulsive treatment—recover after a supervised fast."

What do you eat? is the most neglected question in all of medicine. If more doctors were asking this question and listening sensitively to the answers, the cost of all kinds of illnesses—physical as well as mental— could be reduced.

15.

Who Can Fast—and Who Can't

You should have a thorough physical examination before commencing any fast, even if you feel and look in the best of health. Without such an examination, it is impossible to determine what's going on in the body.

No matter how well you are, you may have some "silent" condition or ailment that would be aggravated by fasting. The blood tests done before the fast serve as a base line from which one monitors the changes occurring during and after the fast.

There are many people who should never fast, and others who should fast only under the closest supervision. You must not fast if you have any of these conditions: heart diseases, especially a predisposition to thrombosis, tumors, bleeding ulcers, cancer, blood diseases, active pulmonary diseases, diabetes (juvenile), gout, liver diseases, kidney diseases, recent myocardial infarction, cerebral diseases.

Any condition requiring long-term use of medication also rules out fasting.

A very thin person can fast, but not for a longer time than one day in a month.

A pregnant woman must not fast, not even for one day. While she herself might tolerate the fast quite well, the developing brain of the fetus might suffer irreparable damage.

A new mother must not fast until her obstetrician has examined her and found that the uterus is back to the pre-pregnant state. For most women this can take more than a month. While nursing, a woman should not fast.

It is perfectly safe for older people to fast, but no older person should *start* fasting without his doctor's approval. There are many elderly people who have been fasting all their lives, and there is considerable evidence that fasting may contribute to a longer life. On the tenth day of a fast, Gandhi at age sixty-four was said to have the constitution of a man of forty. Good-health advocate Bernarr Macfadden discovered fasting in his youth and made it a permanent part of his exceedingly long life. The novelist Upton Sinclair, who lived to be a nonagenarian, found in fasting "a perfect health, a new state of existence, a feeling of purity and happiness," and said that it enabled him to "overwork with impunity." Hygienist and outdoorsman Paul Bragg fasted into his mid-nineties—and was still hiking up and down mountains.

I don't approve of children fasting. It is not known what effect fasting can have on a child's growth processes, and no one should undergo a long fast during years of growth. (I am asked if fasting can help in the treatment of children with learning disabilities. What may help *these* children is a radical change of diet. "Offending foods" make children hyperactive or aggravate hyperactivity caused by something else. In adults they cause fatigue and depression. The elimination of cane sugar and food additives—such as artificial colorings and flavorings and preservatives—helps many children to achieve and learn.)

Among people who *can* fast with great benefit are those with high blood pressure and high cholesterol levels. Abstaining from food can often reduce these readings to normal range. Proper dietary changes can maintain the lowered levels.

High blood pressure should drop progressively during a longer fast. It should remain lower if the weight is kept off. There is a relationship between diabetes and overweight, high blood pressure and high cholesterol. By whatever means weight is lost, lowered blood pressure is the accompanying blessing. By the way, quick weight loss with its correspondingly sudden reduction in blood pressure can bring on feelings of dizziness. Some of these sensations can be averted by avoiding sudden changes in the posture of the body. Rise slowly from a sitting position. Sit up slowly from a lying position. Crouch rather than bend when you pick up something from the floor.

On a longer fast there is a temporary elevation of the cholesterol level. The explanation is that cholesterol deposits "shake loose" and augment the measurable level. But this "increase" is not real; in fact, fasting brings down the level.

Within a week to ten days after the longer fast, the cholesterol level drops to a point much below the prefast level. (The same desirable result is observed when there is loss of weight by any means.) During a long fast, the body chemistry undergoes many beneficial changes. The report one hears about fasting raising cholesterol levels is another of those quarter-truths used by the biased to frighten someone out of undertaking a fast.

There are signs that indicate a fast should be prematurely broken. They usually occur when metabolism is not functioning properly. Persistence of hunger beyond the fourth day, the unexpected return of appetite, persistent irregularity of heartbeat, intestinal spasms, and sustained headaches, vomiting spells, nausea, and dizziness are indications that the fast should be broken and the refeeding program begun. These manifestations are experienced by a small minority of the people who fast.

Hypoglycemics are particularly sensitive to the fasting process on the first day. Blood sugar may drop, and there could be symptoms of weakness, anxiety, and fatigue. If such feelings persist into a second or third day, it would be wise to terminate the fast. Hypoglycemics should fast only under a doctor's *daily* supervison. (Anyone under a doctor's care for any reason should *not* fast, *for even one day*, without approval.)

To repeat: the person in average good health can fast safely for four weeks or longer, but should keep in touch with his or her doctor daily. The long fast must always be a hospital procedure.

16.

Hope for the Young

A herd of mountain sheep in the Canadian province of Alberta is in danger of being killed off by junk food distributed by tourists. The herd eats the candy and other junk food proffered and neglects the normal grass diet. The animals lose weight, and wardens fear females are not producing enough high-quality milk.

Children are fed baby foods spiked with sugar right after they are weaned. They are also fed lollipops and gumdrops by their mothers, fathers, grandparents, their pediatricians, and, so help me, their dentists. Sugar in one form or another is omnipresent in their diet. Little wonder so many of them develop behavioral difficulties, become hyperactive and malnourished, and lack interest in their studies. (The Confectioners Association gave an award to a prominent professor of nutrition for his books and other writings suggesting we'd be better off if we ate *more* sugar and arguing there was nothing wrong with food additives.)

How quickly—and, alas, inevitably—our kids join the fast-food generation! From the moment they get out of bed in the morning, they are besieged on all sides by messages urging them to eat mal-nourishing food. Do they ever hear about the good taste and nutritive values of carrots and sunflower seeds and roasted soybeans? Joan Gussow of Columbia University rightly asked if it were moral to allow our children to be assaulted "with a barrage of food products that add up to audio-visual diabetes." It is distressing to note that the children of the house may be subjected to the nutritional rot of sugar, soft drinks and candy bars and

TV dinners while only the dog of the house rates a balanced diet containing all the essential nutrients.

But there is cheering evidence that a corner is being turned. An encouraging number of young people seem to be acquiring exemplary dietary habits and rejecting the foods hawked to them so persistently in print and electronic advertisements.

In his widely syndicated newspaper column, Sydney J. Harris wrote he wouldn't be surprised if *his* children knew more about nutrition than most doctors do. He said they've studied the subject seriously and have taken vitamin and mineral supplements for years. "The empirical results," he wrote, "are a flowing testimony to their health, strength and endurance."

This knowledge and concern about good eating habits—and I'm sorry to have to concur—does not owe as much as it should to the medical profession, which Mr. Harris points out "is happily writing out millions of prescriptions a month for conditions that would not have existed if proper nutrition had been attended to in the first place."

During a trip West I saw some encouraging evidence of commendable nutritional programs for the young.

President John Howard of Lewis and Clark College, in Portland, who believes the healthy mind needs the support of a healthy body, was concerned the students were being fed a faulty diet. He took action. He ordered a dramatic about-face in the bill of fare. The institutional feeding company servicing the college was told it must develop alternate menus emphasizing natural and nutritious foods.

Among the innovations were buckwheat groats, chop suey made with soybean sprouts, yogurt, vegetable "steaks," granola, toasted wheat germ, cooked whole grains, and fruits and vegetables assembled in tantalizing presentations. Sweet, fatty, highly processed foods were phased out of the students' diet while the nutritional replacements were introduced one at a time so that the switch would not be abrupt. "If I hadn't been told something was up," remarked one student, "I'm not sure I would have noticed the change—except the chow was tasting better and better."

The University of California campus at Santa Cruz developed a student garden project dedicated to organic, ecological horticulture. A young woman, Linda Wilshusen, a graduate of that college, told me the project was designed to "celebrate and foster a true and clear sense of the interdependence of man and his natural environment." She recalled the students ate the food grown in the garden, and that the Whole Earth Restaurant on campus featured such enticing items as pumpkin mushroom soup, lemon-bean salad, brown rice burgers, fresh carrot cake, wheat germ muffins, nut loafs, millet porridge, caraway cabbage salad, whole wheat pasta, and persimmon pudding.

From the other side of the continent came equally good news. The Board of Education of the State of West Virginia unanimously voted a ban on the sale in all public schools of candy, chewing gum, soft drinks, and flavored ice bars. A member of the board said that while it was trying to teach students the value of good nutrition, "there was still available in vending machines food that was bad for them." For those school districts dependent on the profits from vending machines, a list of foods acceptable for vending was compiled. The food included milk, fruit juices, soups, fresh fruits, raisins, peanuts, and yogurt. (As long ago as 1950 this nutritionally progressive state levied a tax on all soft drinks. The money went toward financing West Virginia's University Medical Center in Morgantown.)

The quality of the cuisine began to improve immediately, according to *Prevention* magazine, when innovative Franconia College in New Hampshire discharged its professional catering company and students took over in the cafeteria. (The move to student direction was originally in the interest of cutting expenses.) The students substituted fresh foods for frozen and dried and instant foods. They eliminated white bread and used whole grain bread bought from a local bakery. Yogurt, honey and granola became staples. The soda-vending machine was removed and a soft-drink known as "bug juice" was struck from the menu. By eating better, the students found they were also spending less.

In the Westchester County (New York) town of Hartsdale, a volunteer group of 12 enlightened parents was given authority by the school board to supervise the choice of food served to the 3,500 children in district schools. Eliminated from menus was every food containing artificial colors, flavors and preservatives. The parents substituted whole wheat bread for white bread, decreased the amount of sugar used in recipes, introduced hard-boiled eggs, raisins, sunflower seeds, and a locally baked brand of cookies free of artificial substances. "We are not crazy health food faddists," explained one of the Hartsdale parents. "But it is no more difficult for the vendor to serve nutritious food than overly processed, artificially colored food. Caterers who need our business can be taught to change their ways."

Nutrition is scheduled to be taught from kindergarten through the sixth grade in Hartsdale. A curriculum incorporating the new knowledge about food and its consequences is in the planning stage. Students will learn that orange juice comes from a round, orange-colored fruit and that milk comes from a live cow—not from cartons in a supermarket.

Many of these students may be able to teach the so-called "specialists" a thing or two. Not long ago a university professor of nutrition declared in a press interview that additives were not only *thought* to be safe, but *were* safe—"absolutely. No ifs, ands, or buts." Within a month of the interview, the Food and Drug Administration announced it was moving to ban all further use of the widely applied Red No. 2 on the grounds that it had been shown to cause cancer in laboratory animals.

Good nutritional practices are getting youngsters off to a good start in Allentown, Pennsylvania. The day-care center there run by Volunteers of America has been serving meals of cashew-millet casseroles, brown rice and spinach casseroles, soybean "surprise," and broiled liver. The kids love them. Some of these three-to-five-year-olds come back for seconds and thirds on the liver, which they call "steak." They are also served fresh fruit, mixed raw nuts, seeds, dried fruits, fruited gelatin with yogurt, and homemade whole grain bread. Homemade and natural foods, the Volunteers learned, also cost less than canned and processed foods.

At Bell Top School in North Greenbush, New York, near Albany, candy canes and gumdrops were notably absent from a Christmas party. "The children were not disappointed, they were delighted," reported *Prevention* magazine. "The children had voted unanimously to have only natural goodies that would taste good now and not hurt them later."

Among the hardest misconceptions to quash is the one that eating habits can't be changed or relearned. We have seen that young people's eating preferences *can* be reoriented. A few generations ago, we ate mostly unprocessed or lightly processed foods and we ate at home. More of our food is now industrially prepared and much of it is consumed away from home—and on the run. The consumer advocate Bess Myerson passed along the fact that 80 percent of vending machine sales, which total $6-billion annually, are in junk food categories.

The omens seem favorable that we might be able to re-educate ourselves to the good nutrition—and to the good taste—of our grandparents. It will probably be our children who will lead the way. Already many of them understand that just because it's advertised it is not necessarily good for anyone except the money-oriented processor.

A story in *Fairpress,* a weekly published for residents of Fairfield County, Connecticut, summed up the potential. "Oily French fries, greasy potato chips, filler-packed hot dogs [which contain bone dust and "allowable amounts" of bone splinters]: they're favorites at the beach . . . or are they? Although no one is about to launch a campaign for natural foods to be sold at local public beaches, many people would buy such wholesome items as fresh fruit and fruit juice if they were offered."

At The Door in Manhattan, a "center of alternatives" for troubled youngsters, the kids have crossed out the sign "Candy Shoppe" on the vending machine and written in its place "Food for Thought." Five nights a week some 100 kids dine there on whole and natural foods, which they say have killed their taste for vended junk.

With intelligent eating habits learned early, there would be much less need later for diets—for even "the ultimate diet"—to combat overweight and related ailments.

We will get the food we demand. A nutritionally enlightened public can bring about a revolution in the food industry that can only contribute to the public health.

17.
Sharing and Protesting

Fasting also has altruistic applications.

In effect, the mass fast day can focus concentration on the inequities of food distribution throughout the world—and on a way of alleviating them in some small measure.

Fast days for just such purposes are now organized and nationwide—and increasingly popular. The Thursday before Thanksgiving is taking on the aura of a national holiday. On that day, about a million of us treat our digestive systems to a rest and give the money we would have spent on food for ourselves to support projects that help people in Africa, Asia, and Latin America grow food.

This annual national fast day is sponsored by Oxfam-America, a Boston-headquartered organization dedicated to reminding "thoughtful people of the deepening world food crisis." Pope Paul describes the situation of hunger in the world as "a crisis of solidarity and civilization." The opportunity to convert one day of "hunger" into practical aid for the famished has been hailed as an alternative to inaction, helplessness, and apathy. It is a day of hope.

(And fasting to call attention to the world's hungry is worlds safer than parachuting off the 110-story north tower of the World Trade Center in New York. Which is what Owen Quinn did in 1975. He now confines his appeal to the lecture circuit and leaves the tower to King Kong.)

Oxfam fasts are organized by local educational, religious, civic, and charitable agencies and by individuals. Interest in the event has been stimulated by the participation of such well-known figures as Dr. Benjamin Spock, Senator Richard Clark (of Iowa), Harvard President Derek Bok, the inexhaustible Dick Gregory, and Frances Lappé, the author of *Diet for a Small Planet*. Wisconsinites have been invited to participate by their governor, Patrick Lucy. He proclaimed the fasting day "a chance for us to make a small, personal and significant contribution."

Typical of the enthusiastic responses to national fast days are these comments which Oxfam has shared with us:

"Thank you for providing the structure by which we were able to respond to the world food crisis. . . . The fast focused student attention on this aspect of life with which they were unfamiliar. . . . Thank you for attempting to make us think: think of our bodies, think of our priorities. Thank you for helping me to awaken myself and the people I work with. . . . Everyone in the class who fasted made it through the whole day without eating. It wasn't too difficult and we knew we were not starving. Still, it made us understand a little better what hunger is. . . . If the need for sharing and caring were brought down to a personal level of responsibility all-year-through, we might begin to live more appreciatively by sharing our abundance which rightly belongs to everyone everywhere. . . . We were going out for a pizza when we read about the fast, so we skipped the pizza. Here's the money. . . . We held a foodless food sale and raised $100—the bottles of water went like hotcakes."

Oxfam's Fast for a World Harvest inspired suggestions that such fasts be increased to a once-a-month or even a once-a-week basis.

Between Christmas and New Year's at the end of 1975, Dick Gregory led a week-long fast calling attention to the food shortage in America and in the poor countries of the world. About 120 people joined him at Dr. Ralph Abernathy's Baptist Church in Atlanta. This fast of social protest was endorsed by Stevie Wonder, John Lennon, Eugene McCarthy, Muhammad Ali, Barbra Streisand, and César Chavez. Many people simply can't afford to eat any more, Mr. Gregory contended, pointing out how some have had to take to shoplifting and some to eating dog food. He put forward two proposals: that a new Cabinet post—Secretary of Food and Nutrition—be created and that a new kind of food stamp be issued to guarantee staples like rice, beans, and corn at ten cents a pound.

The prophet Muhammad noted that "the hunger Muslims experience while fasting also enables them to appreciate the hunger of the poor and the needy." Dr. Ahmad H. Sakr, writing in the *Journal of the American Dietetic Association,* suggests that partial fasting could be of some help to politicians "concerned with curbing inflation and energy crises, since people should be able to consume less food and the extra food could be given to those in need. Also, people would have extra time for work, and productivity might be increased."

The individual fast is also employed as an instrument of persuasion. Mahatma Gandhi was the founder in modern times of the protest fast; his inspiring example is being emulated to the present day everywhere in the world.

For example, in righteous indignation over America's underground nuclear tests, a retired professor of ethics, Ichiro Moritaki, has fasted off and on for twenty years before the Cenotaph, the Hiroshima monument containing the names of those killed by the atomic bomb. In the Philippines, a senator, Benigno Aquino, fasted to call attention to the "repressiveness" of the dictatorship of President Marcos. Many individuals fast to protest Soviet repressions.

Commonplace in the United States are hunger strikes in prisons where the inmates are striving to bring about any number of reforms, not the least of which is the deplorable state of the prison diet.

Without for a moment denigrating the aims of Oxfam

and similar organizations and dedicated individuals, the point must be underscored that people who fast to help others and to protest political and social issues are helping themselves at the same time. Any fast is self-serving. One feels better physically as well as mentally, and in the Oxfam context one is entitled to that extra boost in self-regard for "sacrificing" to serve the needs of others.

18.

Fasting Vacations: Retreats and Traveling

One of the laudable fashions of the seventies is the health-improvement vacation.

More and more people are spending vigorous holidays playing tennis, surfing, cross-country skiing, scuba diving, hiking, cycling, mountain climbing, and shooting river rapids.

Others—no less conscientious about their health—are electing to find the true rest and renewal fasting can bring. These people are seeking retreats where fasting and related practices are featured.

A criterion for a fast of any length away from home is the scope of activities available. The more facilities there are, the more involvement, the more quickly time passes, of course.

The best place for a long fast is a spa with facilities for blood analyses, X-rays, electrocardiograms—in other words, a place where examinations are given and the fast is conducted under daily supervision and guidance.

A hospital is the ideal setting for the obese or the seriously ill to fast. Reasonably healthy people should not go to hospitals or to those retreats whose principal concern is in treating serious sickness.

People in good health should avoid the spa where lying in bed is encouraged and where exercise is not part of the daily program. For healthy people, the fasting process is enhanced by exercise.

Fasting and traveling vacations should be compatible, though you rarely see them keeping company. Travel is usually equated with the discovery of new and exotic foods and three-star restaurants.

The most alluring items of any cuisine are always those that are rich or fatty or starchy or sweet. I certainly would not caution a visitor to France to ignore its gastronomic wonders and glorious wines or that in merrye England one should abstain from shepherd's pie, Yorkshire pudding, and strawberry fools. But I do suggest that traveling abroad is an ideal time to fast at least one day a week. (In foreign countries it is a good idea to drink bottled water. This alone puts you into a "fasting situation.") The days you fast give you that much more time—and energy—and money!—to devote to other activities, such as shopping, sight-seeing, and walking around (always good to do while fasting).

One of my correspondents, the peripatetic Lorraine Orr, believes that fasting for a few days *before* trips abroad is an inspired notion for those who can't help traveling on their "stomach." That way, you can approach Europe's groaning boards (if you must!) lean and in good appetite.

Mrs. Orr also suggests fasting might be ideal for coping with jet lag by shortening the time required for our inner clock to synchronize with the time pattern in which we have arrived. (My co-author Jerome Agel fasts in the 24-hour period that includes a trans-Atlantic hop.)

Abroad or home, any time of the year is a good time to fast, but it's preferable where or when temperatures are warm. When no fuel is consumed, the body's thermostat is turned down a few degrees. This is why you are apt to feel chilly when you fast in the winter, even though you are indoors and in a properly heated place.

The temperature outdoors will seem colder than it is; to compensate, you should dress warmly.

One excellent way to keep cool in summer is to fast. Calories generate heat.

19.

Some Often-Asked Questions

In my consultations, lectures, and media interviews around the country, certain questions about fasting recur.

I have prepared a compendium of some of these queries and my answers to them; the answers here incorporate data drawn from current research. (The two questions I'm most frequently asked—How much weight will I lose? and Will I gain back the weight after the fast?—are treated in chapter 5.)

Q.–*What is the difference between "fasting" and "starving"?*

A.–Fasting and starving are entirely different entities. But it is a distinction that eludes many people even in the medical profession; the words can not be used interchangeably. Fasting is a self-rewarding act. Starving is a disaster inflicted upon the hungry by fate or occasionally self-inflicted by the mentally disturbed. During the fast the body is well-nourished from its stored-up "preserves." Starvation begins when the body is deprived of food after the return of appetite. The average overweight person must fast about four weeks before there is return of appetite, which is the signal to break the fast and start eating again. In starvation the body craves food and, being deprived, must consume itself.

Q.–*How does the fasting process keep you from being hungry?*

A.–The body has an automatic device for suppressing

appetite. It is a compound called ketones, the broken-down products of fatty acids. When you fast, the body increases its production of ketones, which are released into the bloodstream. As the amount of ketones increases, appetite is suppressed. The return of appetite is an indication that the fast must be broken. The tongue, which is part of the elimination system, becomes coated and bad breath develops during a longer fast. These symptoms are transitory. They are indications that you are reaping the benefits of the fasting process.

Q.–*Why aren't coffee, tea, and "no-cal" beverages all right during the fast?*

A.–Coffee and tea contain caffeine and tannic acid, respectively. These stimulants excite the central nervous system at a time when the body should be at rest. They add impurities and defeat the cleansing process of the fast. Non-caloric soft drinks "pollute" the body with undesirable chemicals. Their sweet taste—though created artificially, and not by sugar—can arouse stirrings of appetite. The only permissible beverage is water —at least two quarts every day.

Q.–*Are enemas necessary?*

A.–Certainly not on a brief fast. Because they complement and facilitate the fasting process, enemas can be taken every day on the longer fast. *Before* starting a longer fast, it is desirable to take a dose of citrate of magnesia or some other purgative.

Q.–*Don't you overeat after a fast to compensate for "lost meals"?*

A.–One of the prevailing myths is that hunger is cumulative and the satisfaction of hunger only deferred. If you skip 3 meals or 6 meals or 21 meals on a one-day or two-day or a week-long fast—the thinking goes—you will gorge yourself until you've made them up. The truth is, you do *not* accumulate hunger or appetite. One way to guard against overeating after breaking the fast—and this applies to nonfasters as well—is to eat slowly and chew carefully. When you make fasting a way of life, you won't have the urge to overeat.

Q.–*What's happening in fasting research at medical centers?*

A.–A great deal. Important studies have been undertaken in Baltimore, Paris, Cleveland, Moscow, Prague, Stockholm, Houston, Dallas, Los Angeles, São Paulo, Oslo, Brussels, Toronto, Leningrad, Pittsburgh, Philadelphia, Basel, Cork, Turin, Vienna, Dundee, Ghent, Glasgow, Innsbruck, and Palo Alto. Ninety-six doctors and scientists met in Moscow for a week in 1975 to pool their knowledge on "the fasting cure of neurotic and psychiatric patients, patients with skin diseases, and some somatic diseases accompanied by neurotic and mental disturbance." New data were offered to prove the efficiency of the fasting treatment "for treating skin diseases; neurodermatitis; some forms of psoriasis, eczema, gastroenteric diseases, and polyarthritis, provided the fast and re-feeding programs are scrupulously followed." Subjects ranging in age from youngsters to octogenarians, obese and slender, sick and healthy, have been fasted in hospital conditions, in tests lasting from 24 to 33 days, to confirm and extend knowledge of the body's metabolic reactions during fasting. Levels of calcium and potassium rise promptly to normal levels when re-feeding begins. The increasing volume of research on an international "scale" is a hopeful sign the medical profession is recognizing and exploring the use of fasting in the treatment of many human dysfunctions.

Q.–*Can fasting help a chronic underweight problem?*

A.–Paradoxically, the answer is yes, though the question would be better stated, Can you lose weight to gain weight? The point is that food and nutrition are not the same thing. The amount of food taken in is not the key to the state of nutrition; the key is how much food is digested and assimilated. There's considerable evidence fasting helps the chronically underweight person to repair his assimilation functions. Though he may have failed at all previous attempts to gain weight through programs of stepped-up caloric consumption, he will find—when he breaks the fast and starts to eat again—that his food is digested more easily and absorbed more efficiently. He will be eating less than he did before the fast, but finally putting on weight.

Q.–*Can fasting blunt the effects of pollution on the city dweller?*

A.–Urban pollution is now one of the permanent facts of life. We used to think of it as confined principally to cities such as New York and Los Angeles and Pittsburgh and Tokyo. But in my recent travels, I have been appalled to see how the clouds of smog have become nearly ubiquitous, casting their poisonous shadows over such once-"pure" and lovely cities as Phoenix, Mexico City, Denver, and even Palm Springs. The urbanites may not be able to do much about the air they breathe, but a periodic fast cleanses away some of the toxins being absorbed. One of my colleagues believes fasts are *essential* for city dwellers constantly exposed to the exhausts of automobiles, chemicals belched from factory stacks, smoke from incinerators, and—in New York particularly—the gases from tons of dog dung decomposing on the sidewalks and streets.

Q.–*Does fasting turn off the taste for "the good things in life"?*

A.–The "good things in life" relating to food and eating usually mean something sweet, starchy, or alcoholic. Who among us doesn't relish an occasional cocktail or a glass of wine or an indecently rich dessert? These tastes are *not* jeopardized by fasting. As a matter of fact, the brief but regular fast is being used by some people as the way to indulge these tastes without "paying" for it, that is, without gaining weight. One friend told me, "At last I've found a way to have my cakes and ales. . . ." Or, as an amiable Georgian put it, "I don't have to change any of my bad habits. I just put them on ice one day every week." This Southern gentleman likes his bourbon highballs before dinner and such treats at the table as "finger-lickin' good" fried chicken, steaks, candied yams, and pecan pies. I certainly do not recommend items like these as staples in any diet. But if these "good things" are *that* dear to the taste buds, you can go on having them if you stick to a water-only diet one day a week.

Q.–*What is the "protein-sparing fast"?*

A.–Protein-sparing is a medical treatment, not a do-it-yourself regimen. The protein-sparing "fast" is not, strictly speaking, a fast at all; it is a modified or a supplemental fast. Its appeal seems to be to those who still hesitate about the real thing. The erroneous premise of the protein-sparing "fast" is that the total fast is dangerous. If you drink only water, that theory goes, half the weight loss would come out of lean tissues and the result would be a deterioration of muscles, inducing weakness and fatigue and possibly a host of undesirable side effects. While conceding that a total, or real, fast brings about dramatic weight losses, the doctors who devised the supplemental fast contend that protein tissues are "eaten into" concomitantly with fatty tissues when only water is consumed. *This is simply untrue!* The protein supplement comes either in the form of small amounts of lean meat, fish, or fowl, or in a bittersweet formula containing amino acids—components of protein—sometimes mixed with glucose. The meat, fish, or fowl servings may add up to a starvation diet of 700 calories a day; the prescribed amounts of the bittersweet, pre-digested protein formula may amount to 300 calories or more a day. There are reports that the modified fast is easily tolerated and that patients stick to it and achieve weight-loss goals. But the process can be prolonged, requiring daily supervision. My objection to protein-sparing is basic: there is no need for it. It delays and dilutes the benefits of fasting. The body does not begin to consume its lean tissue until the stored-up fat has been utilized. This does not occur before about four weeks of fasting. If overweight is the problem, a true fast will accomplish the loss of weight much more quickly and easily than a modified fast that permits at least 300 calories a day. If the objective is to give the body a complete rest, water alone is preferable to small amounts of food or pre-mixed protein supplements. Anyone who has tried all the fad diets has learned *it is easier to eat nothing at all than to eat reduced rations.* And the personal rewards are much greater. For 5,000 years people have enjoyed fasting without the support of protein-sparing supplements. The promoters of these supplements are trying to board the fasting bandwagon with one foot. By the way, protein-sparing is anything but money-sparing. The treatment is expensive.

Q.–*Can fasting restore virility?*

A.–The claim is made repeatedly that it can, but documentation is hard to come by. Judging from an article in the nation's press, I would say the chance of a man overcoming his infertility through fasting would be promising if he's anything like our simian friends. The article was headlined "Casey's at Bat Again." At the Omaha Zoo a gorilla named Casey was put on a "crash" diet to get his weight down to 420 pounds (from 576). After shaping up, Casey sired a baby. Casey was then a ripe old 20—most gorillas are not potent beyond the ages of 15 to 17. The zoo director also noted that fat animals do not reproduce as well as thin animals. I am also asked if sex is all right during the fast. The answer is that it is more than all right any time both partners are so inclined. Many people, in fact, find both sexual desire and performance enhanced during a fast. Losing weight improves physical appearance, which in turn increases sexual desirability.

Q.–*Can fasting lead to anorexia nervosa?*

A.–Anorexia nervosa is a state of severe emotional disturbance, and often an early symptom of schizophrenia. In my regular practice I have treated many anorexics and in *not a single case* has there been a history of fasting. Here again it is the medical profession at fault for promulgating misinformation and instilling baseless fears. Doctors will warn patients who are perfectly well and emotionally stable that if they fast they may either be unable or unwilling to resume eating; *this is simply untrue.* Any person in average good health does not become anorexic by fasting. Anorexics have a delusion that they are overweight even when they have starved themselves to 80 or so pounds. They alternately starve and gorge themselves. I say "starve" because *they persistently eat small quantities of food* insufficient to support their caloric and nutritional needs. If they eat meat, they broil or fry it until it is almost completely carbonized; in other words, they burn it almost to ashes. Some anorexics have developed the dubious skill of putting a finger deep into their throat to disgorge the food before it has had time to digest and add weight. Some have become so expert at bringing up food they no longer have to use a finger. After gorging, they go to the bathroom or to the kitchen and drink so much water that vomiting is induced. I have never treated an anorexia nervosa who did not have some disturbance of glucose metabolism. A family history of diabetes is also a common finding. Anorexia nervosa is an illness encountered almost exclusively in adolescent girls; only occasionally does a male suffer from it. Anorexics do not fast—they starve.

Q.–*Can fasting induce visions?*

A.–The literature is replete with accounts of visions brought on by fasting. American Indians would placate their gods and "see" a benign fate awaiting them. The Bible tells us Jesus and Moses and Daniel fasted for forty days to bring on divine revelations. The disciples of Eastern mysticism fast in the hope of receiving "other-worldly" illuminations. Extraordinary truths and heavenly messages are said to be received during the extended fast. It is difficult to document this type of phenomenon. Fasts of a day or two or a week induce a tranquil and spiritual feeling, but I personally do not believe mystical visions or celestial revelations are a realistic goal for a fast of any length.

Q.–*Do you recommend the bypass operation, instead of fasting, for the extremely obese?*

A.–I categorically do not recommend the bypass operation, whose purpose is to reduce absorbing surfaces and keep the body from assimilating food. After the operation, patients experience wide mood swings, anxiety, depression, and irritability. Their necessary adjustments in life-style can strain relationships with family and friends. Principal drawbacks of the bypass procedure are the occurrence of major somatic complications, with concomitant discouragement and apprehension, and the fact that benefits may last only two to three years—they are not necessarily permanent. For the extremely obese, fasting in a hospital under supervision is preferable from every point of view.

Q.–*Can pets be fasted?*

A.–Judging from some of the fat cats and plump pooches I see *everywhere* I walk, I would say they most certainly could—and should. (Fasting, as a matter of fact, is routine for animals in the wild and for sick or injured animals.) Just as children become overweight by imitating the eating habits of their overweight parents, overfed pets seem to have masters or mistresses who are overfed. If overstuffed Fanny and petite Fifi can wear matching mink jackets, they surely can join each other in an occasional fast. Whatever Fifi has been eating, by the way, she's been eating better than her master or mistress. The pet food industry seems to lavish far more concern on packaging nutritious fare into those cans of dog and cat food than is expended on products put up for human consumption. J. I. Rodale, founder-publisher of *Prevention* magazine, told of being impressed by the contents on a box he picked up in a supermarket: "Meat and bone meal, ground corn with wheat germ, ground whole wheat with bran and wheat germ, soybean meal, fish meal (including glands and livers), dry milk solids, brewer's yeast, animal fat, cheese meal, sun-dried alfalfa meal, salt, powdered garlic, expertly blended and toasted. . . ." At the bottom of the box it read: "For dogs of discrimination." Mr. Rodale correctly noted that there are many undiscriminating millionaires who are not eating as well.

Q.–How often should you fast for the best results?

A.–Fasting brings many marvelous results. But after years of supervising fasts, I am convinced that an initial fast of whatever length—even as long as a month or until appetite returns—is not sufficient to achieve and sustain *all* the desirable goals. Fasting must become part of the way of life, especially for those who come to it originally to lose weight. It takes more than one fast to secure a revised perspective on the role of food and eating in the life of even the physically and emotionally healthy person. The first fast—regardless of its duration—can be profitably followed by fasting one day a week and one weekend a month. Many people regularly set aside one day every week. (Monday seems to be the most popular time for the one-day-a-week fast, probably to compensate for weekend indulgences.) Some people prefer a three-to-five-day fast once a month. Whatever your pattern of fasting, after an extended fast, it should not exceed a total of six days in a month. A long fast of two consecutive weeks or more should not be repeated for at least six months, and only then in a medical setting. No one should diet or fast himself or herself below the desirable weight for his or her age and height based on medical tables. And remember, no matter how long or how frequently you fast, you should do so only with your doctor's consent.

Q.–*Does fasting prolong the life span?*

A.–Animal studies reported by Susan Seliger in *The National Observer* show that rats fed a low-protein diet one day and then fasted the next day lived 50 percent longer than normally fed rats. Dr. Charles Barrows of the National Institute of Aging discovered that this feeding pattern need not be started from birth. An adult animal put on this regimen will live longer, also. It is widely claimed in the literature that the biological process of aging is slowed by systematic fasting. Herbert Shelton, who directed tens of thousands of fasts, has reported on this phenomenon.

Q.–*If it's said by some to be a "cure-all," why isn't fasting more popular?*

A.–I disagree with the premise that fasting isn't popular. There are millions of "closet" fasters. I am constantly amazed—and pleased—to discover in my travels just how many people throughout the world are "into" fasting. At a dinner party I learned my host and three other guests—all professional people—fast one or two days every week to maintain the weight losses they achieved from a longer fast. Another indication of the growing acceptance of fasting is the widespread media interest. There have been long articles on fasting in high-circulation periodicals like *The New York Times, Town and Country,* the Sunday supplement *Metro, Cosmopolitan, Penthouse-Forum, Playboy,* the *Los Angeles Times, The National Observer,* and *Newsday.* Even *Family Circle,* a supermarket magazine (with a circulation approaching 9,000,000) dependent on food processors for most of its advertising revenue, saw fit to publish a personal-experience feature extolling the virtues of fasting. "Not for Women Only," the nationally syndicated television program moderated by Barbara

Walters and Hugh Downs, did a two-part program on fasting; I was on the panel. Since late 1975 I have discussed fasting on radio and television stations throughout the country and have been interviewed by reporters for some of our most prestigious newspapers and magazines. The increasing worldwide acceptance of fasting makes *Fasting: The Ultimate Diet* an ongoing best seller. I have been informed that fasting retreats here and abroad are doing capacity business and have waiting lists. Fasting will become even *more* "popular" when the myths, fears, and half-truths finally evaporate.

20.

The Joys of Fasting

Fasting is easier than any diet.

Fasting is the quickest way to lose weight.

Fasting can yield weight losses of up to 20 pounds or more in the first week.

Fasting is adaptable to a busy life.

Fasting is used successfully in the treatment of many physical ills.

Fasting gives the body a physiological rest.

Fasting is a calming experience, often relieving tension and insomnia.

Fasting lowers cholesterol and blood-pressure levels.

Fasting frequently induces feelings of euphoria, a natural "high."

Fasting helps to eliminate or modify smoking, drug, and drinking addictions.

Fasting leads to improved dietary habits.

Fasting is a regulator, educating the body to consume only as much food as it needs.

Fasting increases the pleasure of eating.

Fasting produces "found" time—all the hours spent in marketing, preparing, and consuming food and drink.

Fasting is a rejuvenator, slowing the aging process.

Fasting is an energizer, not a debilitator.

Fasting often results in a more vigorous sex life.

Fasting aids in the elimination process.

Fasting rids the body of toxins, giving it an "internal shower."

Fasting does *not* deprive the body of essential nutrients.

Fasting can be used to uncover the sources of food allergies.

Fasting is used effectively in the treatment of schizophrenia and other mental ills.

Fasting under proper supervision can be tolerated easily for anywhere up to four weeks.

Fasting does not accumulate appetite; hunger "pangs" disappear after a day or two.

Fasting is routine for the animal kingdom.

Fasting has been a commonplace experience for man almost as long as he has been eating.

Fasting is a rite in all religions; the Bible alone has 74 references to it.

Fasting under proper conditions is absolutely safe.

Fasting is *not* starving.

Bibliography

Acers, Elva S. Letter to Jerome Agel, May 22, 1976.

Airola, Paavo O. *There Is a Cure for Arthritis.* West Nyack, N.Y.: Parker, 1968.

Allen, Hannah. *The Happy Truth About Protein,* Pearsall, Texas: Healthway Publications.

American Dietetic Association Report. "Position Paper on Food and Nutrition Misinformation on Selected Topics." *Journal of the American Dietetic Association* 66 (3) 1975: 277–80.

Aoki, Thomas T., et al. "Effect of Glucagon on Amino Acid and Nitrogen Metabolism in Fasting Man." *Metabolism: Clinical and Experimental* 23 (9) 1974: 805–14.

———. "Metabolic Effects of Glucose in Brief and Prolonged Fasted Man." *American Journal of Clinical Nutrition* 28 (5) 1975: 507–11.

Arguello, Carlos R. Letters to Jerome Agel, Jan. 30 and March 3, 1976.

Bagdade, J. D., et al. "Basal and Stimulated Hyperinsulinism: Reversible Metabolic Sequelae of Obesity." *Journal of Laboratory and Clinical Medicine* 83 (4) 1974: 563–69.

Balasse, E. O. and Neef, M. A. "Inhibition of Ketogenesis by Ketone Bodies in Fasting Humans." *Metabolism: Clinical and Experimental* 24 (9) 1975: 999–1008.

Ballantyne, F. C., et al. "Albumin Metabolism in Fasting, Obese Subjects." *British Journal of Nutrition* 30 (3) 1973: 585–92.

Barrett, Peter V. D. "Hyperbilirubinemia of Fasting." *Journal of the American Medical Association* 217 (10) 1971: 1349–53.

Benson, J. W. Jr., et al. "Glucose Utilization by Sweat Glands During Fasting in Man." *Journal of Investigative Dermatology* 63 (3) 1974: 287–91.

Berman, Steve. "Fasting: An Old Cure for Fat, A New Treatment for Schizophrenia." *Prevention,* Jan. 1976: 27–31.

Blackburn, George L. Letter to Jerome Agel, March 4, 1976.

Blackburn, George L., et al. "Protein Sparing Therapy During

Periods of Starvation with Sepsis or Trauma." *Annals of Surgery* 177 (5) 1973: 588–94.

Block, Marshall B. "Hypoglycemia: Clinical Implications. Part II: Fasting Hypoglycemia." *Arizona Medicine* 32 (1) 1975: 37–39.

Bolzano, K., et al. "Effect of Total Starvation on Cardiac Output of Overweight Women with Normal Circulation." *Wiener Klinische Wochenschrift* 85 (40) 1973: 657–61.

Boulter, Philip R. Letter to Jerome Agel, May 24, 1976.

Boulter, Philip R., et al. "Dissociation of the Renin-Aldosterone System and Refractoriness to the Sodium-Retaining Action of Mineralocorticoid During Starvation in Man." *Journal of Clinical Endocrinology and Metabolism* 38 (2) 1974: 248–54.

————. "Effect of Aldosterone Blockade During Fasting and Refeeding." *American Journal of Clinical Nutrition* 26 (April) 1973: 397–402.

————. "Pattern of Sodium Excretion Accompanying Starvation." *Metabolism: Clinical and Experimental* 22 (5) 1973: 675–82.

Bricklin, Mark. "Color His Face Red 2." *Prevention,* April 1976: 78.

Brodie, Franklin. Letter to the Editor, *The New York Times Magazine,* Dec. 15, 1974: 35.

Brody, Jane E. "Additional Evidence Indicates That Diet Is a Cancer Cause." *The New York Times,* Dec. 2, 1975: 1+.

Brosius, Dorothy K. Letter to Jerome Agel. (undated)

Burros, Marian. "Our Food: Refined Way to Die?" *The Washington Post,* Oct. 23, 1975.

————. "Pet Food: A Dietary Staple for Impoverished Americans." *The Washington Post,* Dec. 7, 1975: D2.

Busse Grawitz, P. Letter to Jerome Agel (undated).

Cady, Steve. "Olympic Diet: Hold the Steak, Vitamins." *The New York Times,* June 11, 1976: D13+.

Cahill, Kathleen. Letter to Jerome Agel from Oxfam-America, Dec. 6, 1976.

Calloway, Doris Howes. "Recommended Dietary Allowances for Protein and Energy." *Journal of the American Dietetic Association* 64 (Feb.) 1974: 157–62.

Carter, Michelle. "Try Fasting for Weight Control." *San Mateo* (Calif.) *Times,* Sept. 30, 1975.

Carter, William J., et al. "Effect of Thyroid Hormone on Metabolic Adaptation to Fasting." *Metabolism: Clinical and Experimental* 24 (10) 1975: 1175–83.

Cerra, Frances. "Parents Close Top on Sodas in Westchester School Menu." *The New York Times,* Feb. 3, 1976: 33.

Chandler, Russell. "A Life of Freedom in 'Voluntary Poverty,'" *The Washington Post,* Dec. 14, 1975: D2.

Chandler, Stephen T. Letter to Allan Cott, June 18, 1975.

Chaussain, J. L. Letter to Jerome Agel, April 7, 1976.

————. "Glycemic Response to 24-Hour Fast in Normal Children and Children with Ketotic Hypoglycemia." *Journal of Pediatrics* 82 (3) 1973: 438–43.

Chaussain, J. L., et al. "Effect of Fast in Normal Children: Influence of Age." Unpublished paper.

————. "Effect of 24-Hour Fast in Obese Children." Unpublished paper.

————. "Glycemic Response to 24-Hour Fast in Normal Children and Children with Ketotic Hypoglycemia: II. Hormonal and Metabolic Changes." *Journal of Pediatrics* 85 (6) 1974: 776–81.

Cheatham, R. J. Letter to Jerome Agel, May 14, 1976.

Cherry, Rona. "McDonald's Goes to School in Arkansas." *The New York Times*, Sept. 30, 1976.

Chesney, Peter J. "Tyringham Naturopathic Clinic." Reprinted from *Here's Health*.

Christophe, A. Letters to Jerome Agel, June 9 and Sept. 23, 1976.

Christophe, A. and Verdonk, G. "Effect of Prolonged Fasting on Serum Lipids and Serum Lipo-proteins in Obese Men." *Hoppe-Seyler's Zeitschrift für Physiologische Chemii* 355 (10) 1974: 1184.

Cincinnati Enquirer, The. "Well-Padded Women Belie Diet, Spa Fads." June 1, 1976: 1.

Clancy, Mary Louise. "Fasting Gains New-Found Popularity." *Twin Circle*, Dec. 14, 1975.

Clark, Michael. "Franconia, Maybe What a College Ought to Be. *Prevention*, August 1976.

Clements, F. W. "Nutrition 11: Recommended Dietary Allowances." *Medical Journal of Australia* 62–2 (1) 1975: 24–26.

Cockburn, Alexander and Ridgeway, James. "The Greasy Pole." *The Village Voice*, May 31, 1976.

Committee on Nutritional Misinformation. "Vegetarian Diets." National Academy of Sciences, May 1974.

Conners, Bernard F. *Don't Embarrass the Bureau.* New York: Avon, 1973.

Cooper, Donald L., with Fair, Jeff. "Pregame Meal: To Eat or Not to Eat—and What?" *The Physician and Sportsmedicine*, Nov. 1975.

Costill, David L. Letter to Jerome Agel, Nov. 2, 1976.

Cott, Allan with Agel, Jerome and Boe, Eugene. *Fasting: The Ultimate Diet.* New York: Bantam, 1975.

Cott, Allan. "Controlled Fasting Treatment for Schizophrenia." *The Journal of Orthomolecular Psychiatry* 3 (4) 1974: 301–11.

Cravetto, C. A., et al. "Metabolic Aspects of Prolonged Fasting in Obese Subjects." *Folia Endocrinologica* 26 (2) 1973: 139–52.

Crosby, William H. "Can a Vegetarian Be Well Nourished?" *Journal of the American Medical Association* 233 (8) 1975: 898.

Damon, G. Edward. "A Primer on Dietary Minerals." *FDA Consumer,* Sept. 1974.

————. "A Primer on Food Additives." *FDA Consumer,* May 1973.

————. "A Primer on Four Nutrients: Proteins, Carbohydrates Fats, and Fiber." *FDA Consumer,* Feb. 1975.

Davis, Gwen. Letter to Jerome Agel, March 22, 1976.

de Saumarez, Lady Julia. Letters to Jerome Agel, March 17 and April 13, 1976.

Dept. of Health, Education and Welfare. Letter to Jerome Agel, Sept. 3, 1976.

Dosti, Rose. "Fasting? See Your Doctor." *Los Angeles Times,* Nov. 13, 1975: IV,1.

Dougherty, Paul, "High-Speed Juice Diet Helps Star Man Lose 12 Lbs. in Just Six Days." *The Star,* June 8, 1976: 9.

Downs, Hugh. Letter to Jerome Agel, March 1, 1976.

Drenick, E. J., et al. "Energy Expenditure in Fasting Obese Men." *Journal of Laboratory and Clinical Medicine* 81 (3) 1973: 421–30.

Duran, Mary. "Fasting Improves Health." *Atlantic City* (N.J.) *Press,* Sept. 7, 1975.

Dusky, Lorraine. "Fasting on the Run." *Town and Country,* July 1975.

Dwyer, Johanna. "Protein: Why You Need It. Where You Get It." *Redbook* 144 (March) 1975: 85+.

Dwyer, Johanna, et al. "The New Vegetarians: The Natural High?" *Journal of the American Dietetic Association* 65 (Nov.) 1974: 529–36.

Erhard, Darla. "Nutrition Education for the 'Now' Generation." *Journal of Nutrition Education* 2 (4) 1971: 135–39.

Ettenberg, Selma. Letter to Jerome Agel (undated).

Ewald, Ellen Buchman. *Recipes for a Small Planet.* New York: Ballantine, 1973.

Fineberg, Seymour K. "The Realities of Obesity and Fad Diets." *Nutrition Today,* July/Aug. 1972: 23.

Fleming, Laura W. and Stewart, W. K. "Effect of Carbohydrate Intake on the Urinary Excretion of Magnesium, Calcium, and Sodium in Fasting Obese Patients," *Nephron* 16 (1) 1976: 64–73.

Fogel, Suzanne. Letter to Jerome Agel, June 1, 1976.

Food for Fitness. Mt. View, Calif.: World Publications, 1975.

Forbes, Gilbert B. "Weight Loss During Fasting: Implications for the Obese." *The American Journal of Clinical Nutrition* 23 (9) 1970: 1212–19.

Ford, Norman. "I Travel for Health." *Prevention,* June 1976: 94–101.

————. Letters to Jerome Agel, May 15 and June 6, 1976.

Fremon, David. "Fasting for Fun and Peril." *Chicago Sun-Times Midwest Magazine,* June 8, 1975: 15–16.

Freour, P., et al. "Blood Alcohol and the Consumption of Alcoholic Beverages Fasting and During a Meal." *Revue d'Epidémiologie Médecine Sociale et Santé Publique* 20 (8) 1972: 757–71.

Friggens, Paul. "The Corn That Could Change the Lives of Millions." *Reader's Digest* 106 (633) 1975: 144–48.

Fry, T. C. *Program for Dynamic Health.* Chicago: Natural Hygiene Press, 1974.

————. *Superior Foods, Diet Principles and Practices for Perfect Health.* Pearsall, Texas: Healthway Publications.

Gedde-Dahl, D. "Fasting Serum Gastrin Levels in Humans with Low Pentagastrin-Stimulated Gastric Acid Secretion." *Scandinavian Journal of Gastroenterology* 9 (6) 1974: 597–99.

Gelman, A., et al. "Role of Metabolic Acidosis on Renal Function During Starvation." *American Journal of the Medical Sciences* 266 (1) 1973: 33–36.

Genuth, Saul M., et al. "Weight Reduction in Obesity by Outpatient Semistarvation." *Journal of the American Medical Association* 230 (7) 1974: 987–91.

Gilbert, C. H. and Galton, D. J. "The Effect of Catecholamines and Fasting on Cyclic-AMP and Release of Glycerol from Human Adipose Tissues." *Hormone and Metabolic Research* 6 (3) 1974: 229–33.

Glasser, Ronald J. "Being a Medical Hero Can Be Hell" (excerpt from *The Body Is the Hero*). *Prevention,* May 1976: 70–76.

Goeschke, H. and Lauffenburger, T. "Breath Acetone and Ketone in Normal and Overweight Subjects During Total Fasting." *Research in Experimental Medicine* 165 (3) 1975: 233–44.

Goeschke, H., et al. "Nitrogen Loss in Normal and Obese Subjects During Total Fast." *Klinische Wochenschrift* 53 (13) 1975: 605–10.

Good Housekeeping Institute. "Foods That Give the Most Protein for Your Money." *Good Housekeeping* 179 (Nov.) 1974: 244+.

Gordon, John Steele. Letter to the Editor, *The New York Times Magazine,* Dec. 15, 1974: 35.

Gravenhorst, A. G. Letter to Jerome Agel, Feb. 24, 1976.

Graydon, J. Graeme. Letter to Jerome Agel, May 25, 1976.

Greenblatt, David J., et al. "Bioavailability of Digoxin Tablets and Elixir in the Fasting and Postprandial States." *Clinical Pharmacology and Therapeutics* 16 (3, Part I) 1974: 444–48.

Grotta-Kurska, Daniel. "Before You Say 'Baloney' . . . Here's What You Should Know About Vegetarianism." *Today's Health* 52 (10) 1974: 18+.

———. "Do We Eat Too Much Meat?" *Reader's Digest* 106 (634) 1975: 195–200.

Gussow, Joan. Conversation with Eugene Boe, June 1, 1976.

Halperin, Mitchell L., et al. "Effects of Fasting on the Control of Fatty-Acid Synthesis in Hepatoma 777 and Host Liver: Role of Long-Chain Fatty Acyl-COA, the Metochondrial Citrate Transporter and Pyruvate Behydrogenase Activity." *European Journal of Biochemistry* 50 (3) 1975: 517–22.

Hammer, Leon I. Letter to Jerome Agel, May 20, 1976.

Hansen, A. and Weeke, J. "Fasting Serum Growth Hormone Levels and Growth Hormone Responses in Exercise During Normal Menstrual Cycles and Cycles of Oral Contraceptives." *Scandinavian Journal of Clinical and Laboratory Investigation* 34 (3) 1974: 199–205.

Hardinge, Mervyn G. "Raising Infant on Vegetarian Diet." Questions and Answers, *Journal of the American Medical Association* 227 (1) 1974: 88.

Hardinge, Mervyn G. and Crooks, Hulda. "Non-Flesh Dietaries." *Journal of the American Dietetic Association* 43 (6) 1963: 545–58.

Hardinge, Mervyn G. and Stare, Frederick J. "Nutritional Studies of Vegetarians." *The Journal of Clinical Nutrition* 2 (2) 1954: 73–88.

Harper's Weekly. "Mac the Knife." May 31, 1976.

"Health Hydros and Farms in England." English Tourist Board, Information 12.

Hedner, Pavo, et al. "Insulin Release in Fasting Man Induced by Impure but Not by Pure Preparations of Cholecystokinin." *ACTA Medica Scandinavica* 97 (1–2) 1975: 109–112.

Heesen, H., et al. "Thiamin and Thiamin Pyrophosphate in Obese Patients on Reducing Diet and Complete Fasting." *Deutsche Medizinische Wochenschrift* 100 (11) 1975: 544–48.

Heyden, S., et al. "Weight Reduction in Adolescents." *Nutrition and Metabolism* 15 (4/5) 1973: 295–304.

Hill, John W. Letter to Jerome Agel, May 7, 1976.

Hoffer, A. Review of *Fasting: The Ultimate Diet*, 1976.

Hurst, Lynda. "How You Can Lose Weight Fast." *Toronto Star*, Oct. 30, 1976: F-1.

Illich, Ivan. *Medical Nemesis.* New York: Pantheon, 1976.

James, George. " '75 High Jumper Falls Free." *New York News*, July 23, 1976: 5.

Jones, J. J. and Gelfand, M. "Fasting Serum Lipoproteins in Rural Africans in Rhodesia, Measured by Filtration and Nephelometry." *Clinica Chimica ACTA* 57 (2) 1974: 131–34.

Journal of the American Dietetic Association. "Obesity and Unemployment." 65 (Feb.) 1974: 162.

————. "Vegetarian Diets." 65 (Aug.) 1974: 121–22.

Journal of the American Medical Association. "Obesity: A Continuing Enigma." 211 (3) 1970: 493.

Kalkhoff, R. K. and Kim, H. J. "Metabolic Responses to Fasting and Ethanol Infusion in Obese Diabetic Subjects. Relationship to Insulin Deficiency." *Diabetes* 22 (5) 1973: 372–80.

Kinderlehrer, Jane. "Students Do Better with A-Plus Food." *Prevention,* June 1976: 70–73.

Kirban, Salem. *How to Keep Healthy and Happy by Fasting.* Huntingdon Valley, Penna.: Salem Kirban Inc., 1976.

Kolanowski, J., et al. "Further Evaluation of the Role of Insulin in Sodium Retention Associated with Carbohydrate Administration after a Fast in the Obese." *European Journal of Clinical Investigation* (2) 1972: 439–44.

————. "Hormonal Adaptation to Short-Term Total Fast in the Obese." *Médecin et Hygiène* 1975: 112–16.

————. "Influence of Fasting on Adrenocortical and Pancreatic Islet Response to Glucose Loads in the Obese." *European Journal of Clinical Investigation* (1) 1970: 25–31.

————. "Influence of Glucagon on Sodium (Na) Balance During Fasting and Carbohydrate Refeeding in the Obese." *European Journal of Clinical Investigation* in *European Society for Clinical Investigation Abstracts* 3 (3) 1973: 244–45.

————. "Metabolic and Hormonal Effects of Short-Term Total Starvation in Obesity." *Schweizerische Medizinische Wochenschrift* 104 (29) 1974: 1022–28.

————. "Sodium Balance and Renal Tubular Sensitivity to Aldosterone During Total Fast and Carbohydrate Refeeding in the Obese." *European Journal of Clinical Investigation* (6) 1976: 75–83.

Kolata, G. B. "Brain Biochemistry: Effects of Diet." *Science* 192 (Apr. 2) 1976: 41–42.

Kuhn, E. "Renal Response to a Water Load in Normal Fasting Subjects." *Nutrition and Metabolism* 16 (3) 1974: 163–71.

Ladies Home Journal. "The Main Course Takes New Course: Lots to Eat Without the Meat." 91 (March) 1974: 86+.

Lanza, Karen. Letter to Jerome Agel, May 19, 1976.

Lappé, Frances Moore. *Diet for a Small Planet.* New York: Ballantine, 1971.

Leigh, Robin. "Fasting: The Ultimate Diet," a review, *Sun Reporter,* Sept. 20, 1975.

Leighty, John M. "The Many Benefits of Fasting." *Newhall* (Calif.) *Signal,* Nov. 12, 1975.

Levick, Diane. "Junk Food Junkies Could Kick Habit at Beach." *Fairpress* (Westport, Conn.), July 14, 1976: 4a.

Lewis, George. Letter to Allan Cott, Aug. 6, 1975.

————. Letter to Jerome Agel, March 10, 1976.

Lewis, Harold. "The Sure Way to Lose Weight—When All Else Fails." *National Enquirer,* Oct. 26, 1975.

Lilly, John C. Letter to Jerome Agel, June 1, 1976.

Liporetskii, B. M. and Ryzhov, V. M. "Changes in Free Fatty Acid Levels and Triglyceride in Blood After Fasting and Food Loads in the Assessing Lipid Metabolism in Patients with Atherosclerosis." *Kardiologiya* 14 (5) 1974: 40–43.

Love, Sam. "A Delicious Collection of Essays for the 'Real Food' Movement." *The Washington Post,* Oct. 16, 1976: B-2.

MacFadyen, U. M., et al. "Starvation and Human Slow-Wave Sleep." *Journal of Applied Physiology* 35 (3) 1973: 391–94.

McKinney, Joan. "It's a Fast Way to Lose That Weight." *Oakland* (Calif.) *Tribune,* Aug. 29, 1975: 30.

Majumder, Sanat K. "Vegetarianism: Fad, Faith or Fact." *American Scientist* 60, 1972: 175–179.

Mann, George V. "Raising Infant on Vegetarian Diet," Questions and Answers, *Journal of the American Medical Association* 227 (1) 1974: 88.

Marks, Marjorie. "This Door Leads to Better Food for Teens." *Prevention,* Dec. 1976: 142.

Mayer, Jean. "The Practical Way to Learn." *The Washington Post,* Oct. 23, 1975: D6.

Mayer, Jean and Dwyer, Johanna. "Vegetarianism—Healthy Way of Life." *New York News,* Dec. 8, 1976: 58.

Maynard, Joyce. "Abstinence Without Tears." *The New York Times,* Nov. 10, 1976.

Mehta, Ved. "Mahatma Gandhi and His Apostles," Part II. *The New Yorker,* May 17, 1976.

Mercer, Marilyn. "More Protein for Your Money." *McCall's,* Feb. 1975: 43.

Merimee, T. J. and Tyson, John E. "Stabilization of Plasma Glucose During Fasting." *New England Journal of Medicine* 291 (24) 1974: 1275–78.

Miller, D. S. and Payne, P. R. "Weight Maintenance and Food Intake." *Journal of Nutrition* 78, 1962: 255–62.

Miller, Don Ethan. "How I Tried to Fast for a Week and Lived." *The Village Voice,* May 3, 1976: 27.

Miller, James C. Letter to Jerome Agel.

Minneapolis Tribune. "Looking Back on Being Raised as a Lady." May 30, 1976.

Moore, John G. Letter to Jerome Agel, May 10, 1976.

Moore, William. "Brown's Strange Eating Habits." *San Francisco Chronicle,* March 5, 1976: 1+.

————. Letter to Jerome Agel, June 11, 1976.

Myerson, Bess. "How to Beat Junk Food 'Machine.'" *New York News,* Aug. 4, 1976.

National Catholic Welfare Conference. *Poenitemini: Apostolic Constitution on Fast and Abstinence.* Feb. 17, 1966.

National Dairy Council. "Health Implications of Fad Reducing Diets." *Dairy Council Digest* 37 (2) 1966: 7–10.

"NBC Reports: What Is This Thing Called Food?" Sept. 8, 1976.

Nelson, Ralph A. "What Should Athletes Eat? Unmixing Folly and Facts." *The Physician and Sportsmedicine,* Nov. 1975: 67–72.

New Times. "The Diet that Drives You to Drink." April 1, 1976: 20.

New York News. "Caroline Hit by Disorder of the Stomach." April 30, 1976.

———. "Casey's at Bat Again." Feb. 11, 1976.

———. "Gilmore Will Get His 3rd Date With Death." Dec. 15, 1976.

New York Times, The. "Is Travel Really Broadening?" Feb. 15, 1976: VII, 1.

———. "New Scale Can Detect Bite-Sized Weight Gain." June 4, 1976.

New Yorker, The. "Talk of the Town: Fast." Jan. 19, 1976: 21–22.

———. May 17, 1976. p. 120.

News (Mexico City). "Doctor Welch." March 5, 1976: 18.

Nicolayev, Yuri. Letters to Jerome Agel, April 22 and May 6, 1976.

———. Summary of Conference at Moscow Psychiatric Institute on Fasting Cure, May 13–15, 1975.

Nicolayev, Yuri and Rudakov, Y. Y. "Psychobiological Training of Human Regulatory Protective and Adaptive Mechanisms." *Biologie Aviakosm Medicine* 9 (1) 1975: 86–88.

Nilsson, L. H. and Hultman, E. "Liver Glycogen in Man—the Effect of Total Starvation or a Carbohydrate-Poor Diet Followed by Carbohydrate Refeeding." *Scandinavian Journal of Clinical and Laboratory Investigation* 32 (4) 1973: 325–30.

North, K. A. K., et al. "The Mechanisms by Which Sodium Excretion Is Increased During a Fast but Reduced on Subsequent Carbohydrate Feeding." *Clinical Science and Molecular Medicine* 46 (4) 1974: 423–32.

Not For Women Only. "Fasting/Dieting/Eating," television syndicated series.

Novich, Max M. Letter to Jerome Agel, April 20, 1976.

Null, Gary. "Fasting." *Let's Live,* Nov. 1975: 84–89.

Null, Gary and Staff. *The Complete Question and Answer Book of General Nutrition.* New York: Dell, 1974.

Nutrition Reviews. "FAO/WHO Handbook on Human Nutritional Requirements, 1974." 33 (5) 1975: 147–51.

———. "Fasting for Obese Children." 26 (11) 1968: 335–36.

———. "Food Faddism." 32 (Supplement) 1974: 53.

O'Connell, R. C. "Nitrogen Conservation in Starvation: Graded Responses to Intravenous Glucose." *Journal of Clinical Endocrinology and Metabolism* 39 (3) 1974: 555–63.

Oles, Michael. Letter to the Editor, *The Village Voice,* May 17, 1976: 6.

Orr, Lorraine. Letter to Jerome Agel, 1976.

Oxfamnews. "Fast for a World Harvest Gives U.S. a Taste of Hunger." 1 (1) 1975: 1+.

———. "Oxfam's Nov. 20 Fast Focuses National Spotlight on Hunger." 2 (1) 1976.

Parrish, John B. "Implications of Changing Food Habits for Nutrition Educators." *Journal of Nutrition Education* 2 (4) 1971: 140–46.

Perry, Jean. "Bottled Water Floods Market." *New York News,* Oct. 19, 1976: 39.

Physical Culture. 85 (5) 1941: 57.

———. 85 (6) 1941: 4–5.

Pines, Maya. "Meatless, Guiltless." *The New York Times Magazine,* Nov. 24, 1974: 48+.

Pinsof, Barbara. Letter to Jerome Agel, April 11, 1976.

Porter, Sylvia. "Monitoring School Meals." *New York Post,* April 29, 1976: 30.

Prevention. "A Holistic Coach." June 1976: 93.

———. "Junk Food Is More than a Bad Joke." Oct. 1976: 80.

———. "J. I. Rodale Said It." May 1976: 77.

———. "Let's Give Our Children a Taste of Honest Food (For a Change!)." May 1976: 127+.

———. "Upgrading School Lunches—One Town's Response." Oct. 1976: 12.

———. "West Virginia Expels Junk Food From Public Schools." April 1976: 91.

———. Feb 1976: 92 and 179.

———. April 1976: 146.

Randal, Judith. "Fat-Stuffed Diets Are Panned as Factor in Cancer." *New York News,* Dec. 12, 1976: 16.

Raper, Nancy R. and Hill, Mary M. "Vegetarian Diets." *Nutrition Program News,* U.S. Department of Agriculture, July/Aug. 1973.

Raskin, Philip, et al. "Effect of Insulin Glucose Infusions on Plasma Glucagon Levels in Fasting Diabetics and Non-Diabetics." *Journal of Clinical Investigation* 56 (5) 1975: 1132–38.

Rath, R. and Masek, J. "Changes in the Nitrogen Metabolism in Obese Women after Fasting and Refeeding." *Metabolism: Clinical and Experimental* 15 (1) 1966: 1–8.

Rath, R., et al. "Catecholamines and Obesity, Fasting and the Adrenergic System." *Endokrinologie* 62 (2) 1973: 225–33.

————. "Relationship of Lipid and Carbohydrate Metabolism in Women During Fasting." *Review of Czechoslovak Medicine* 13 (4) 1967: 231–37.

Register, U. D. and Sonnenberg, L. M. "The Vegetarian Diet." *Journal of the American Dietetic Association* 62 (3) 1973: 253–61.

Rensberger, Boyce. "Nutrition Panel Urges Studies to Spur Production of Protein." *The New York Times,* Dec. 20, 1975: 30.

Romney, George. Letter to Jerome Agel, June 12, 1976.

Rosenbaum, Ken. "Overeaters, Here's Fast, Fast Relief." *Cleveland Press,* Sept. 26, 1975: 27.

Ross, Shirley. *Fasting.* New York: St. Martin's, 1975.

Runcie, J. and Hilditch, T. E. "Energy Provision, Tissue Utilization, and Weight Loss in Prolonged Starvation." *British Medical Journal* 2 (5915) 1974: 352–56.

Runner's World Magazine. "The Runner's Diet." Booklet of the Month, No. 14, 1972.

Sakr, Ahmad. "Fasting in Islam." *Journal of the American Dietetic Association* 67 (1) 1975: 17–21.

San Francisco Examiner. Feb. 27, 1976: 19.

Sanders, Mary Jane. "Voluntary Fasting Cures Many Ills." *Post-Tribune* (Gary, Ind.), Sept. 5, 1975.

Sapir, D. G. and Owen, O. E. "Renal Conservation of Ketone Bodies During Starvation." *Metabolism: Clinical and Experimental* 24 (1) 1975: 23–33.

Sapir, D. G., et al. "Nitrogen Sparing Induced by a Mixture of Essential Amino Acids Given Chiefly as Their Keto-Analogues During Prolonged Starvation in Obese Subjects." *Journal of Clinical Investigation* 54 (4) 1974: 974–80.

Sassoon, Beverly and Vidal. *A Year of Beauty and Health.* New York: Simon and Schuster, 1975.

Saudek, C. D., et al. "The Natriuretic Effect of Glucagon and Its Role in Starvation." *Journal of Clinical Endocrinology and Metabolism* 36 (4) 1973: 761–65.

Sauer, Georgia. "Lose Weight, Not Shirt: A Guide to Nearby Reducing Spas." *New York Sunday News,* May 16, 1976: 31+.

Schlick, W., et al. "Energy Exchange During Total Starvation." *Medizin und Ernährung* 13 (10) 1972: 215–20.

Seiberling, Dorothy. "The Art-Martyr." *New York,* May 24, 1976.

Selinger, Susan. "Fasting: An Idea to Chew On." *The National Observer,* Dec. 11, 1976: 1.

Seventeen. "Breakfast of Champions?" April 1976: 170+.

Shelton, Herbert M. *Fasting Can Save Your Life.* Chicago: Natural Hygiene Press, 1964.

————. *Fasting for Renewal of Life.* Chicago: Natural Hygiene Press, 1974.

————. *Food Combining . . . Made Easy* (Dr. Shelton's Health School).

Sidhwa, Keki R. Letters to Jerome Agel, March 20 and April 5, 1976.

Sigler, M. H. "The Mechanism of the Natriuresis of Fasting." *Journal of Clinical Investigation* 55 (2) 1975: 377–87.

Silverstein, Philip. Letter to Allan Cott, Aug. 20, 1975.

————. Letter to Jerome Agel. (undated)

Slany, J., et al. "Cardiovascular Effects of Starvation in Obese Subjects." *Wiener Klinische Wochenschrift* 86 (15) 1974: 423–28.

Spahn, U. and Plenert, W. "Changes in the Body Composition of Obese Children During Absolute Starvation." *Zeitschrift für Kinderheilkunde* 115 (1) 1973: 59–69.

Spahn, U., et al. "Changes in Parameters Appertaining to Lipolysis in Obese Children during a Weight-Reducing Regimen." *Zeitschrift für Kinderheilkunde* 114, 1973: 131–42.

Spark, Richard F. Letter to Jerome Agel, April 28, 1976.

Spark, Richard F., et al. "Renin, Aldosterone and Glucagon in the Natriuresis of Fasting." *New England Journal of Medicine* 292 (June 19) 1975: 1335–40.

Spitze, Hazel Taylor. "Innovative Techniques for Teaching Nutrition." *Journal of Nutrition Education* 2 (4) 1971: 156–58.

Steinman, Marion. "Beauty: From the Inside Out." *The New York Times Magazine*, Feb. 29, 1976: 60+.

Stephenson, Marilyn. "Making Food Labels More Informative." *FDA Consumer*, Sept. 1974.

Stern, Judith S. "How to Stay Well on a Vegetarian Diet and Save Money Too!" *Vogue* 165 (Feb.) 1975: 151.

Stewart, W. K. and Fleming, L. W. "Relationship Between Plasma and Erythrocyte Magnesium and Potassium Concentrations in Fasting Obese Subjects." *Metabolism: Clinical and Experimental* 22 (4) 1973: 535–47.

Stinebaugh, Bobby J. "Taste Thresholds for Salt in Fasting Patients." *American Journal of Clinical Nutrition* 28 (8) 1975: 814–17.

Stone, Sebastian. Letter to Jerome Agel, 1976.

Stry, David. Letter to Jerome Agel, March 5, 1976.

Stuckey, William K. "The 'No-Aging Diet': Something Fishy Here." *New York*, Oct. 11, 1976: 73.

Stunkard, Albert J. and Rush, John. "Dieting and Depression Re-examined: A Critical Review of Untoward Responses During Weight Reduction for Obesity." *Annals of Internal Medicine* 81 (4) 1974: 526–33.

Taylor, Henry Longstreet, et al. "The Effects of Successive Fasts on the Ability of Men to Withstand Fasting During Hard Work." *American Journal of Physiology* 143 (1) 1945: 148–55.

Thornton, Kellen C. "Steak, Too, Can Be 'Junk Food,'" *Fergus Falls* (Minn.) *Journal*, July 28, 1976.

Thornton, William M. Letter to Allan Cott, Aug. 23, 1975.

———. Letter to Jerome Agel, April 20, 1976.

Time. "Dieting by Starving." Nov. 22, 1976: 53.

———. "The Joy of Aging." Nov. 8, 1976: 86.

Tom, Gail and Rucker, Margaret. "Fat, Full, and Happy: Effects of Food Deprivation, External Cues, and Obesity on Preference Ratings, Consumption, and Buying Intentions." *Journal of Personality and Social Psychology* 32 (5) 1975: 761–66.

Trask, Debra. Letter and Data to Eugene Boe, Oct. 1, 1976.

Trecker, Barbara. "Fasting: A Dangerous Diet?" *New York Post,* April 26, 1975.

Trenchard, P. M. and Jennings, R. D. "Diurnal Variation in Glucose Tolerance and Its Reversal by Lengthened Fasting." *British Medical Journal* 2 (5920) 1974: 640–42.

Ubell, Earl. "Hyperkinesis: Pep Pills to Quiet the Over-Peppy Child." *The New York Times,* March 14, 1971.

Unger, Andrew. "Fasting: A Fast Way to Lose—If You Can Stomach It." *Moneysworth,* Jan. 1976.

United States Catholic Conference. *Our Daily Bread, Vol. II.* Sept. 1975.

United States Department of Health, Education and Welfare. *Obesity and Health,* Chapter 7: "Treatment Guidelines for Successful Treatment."

United States Departments of Agriculture and Health, Education and Welfare. "Food Is More Than Just Something to Eat."

Van Lear, Denise. "Come Fast With Me," a fasting account submitted to Jerome Agel, May 8, 1976.

Vidalon, C., et al. "Age-related Changes in Growth Hormone in Non-diabetic Women." *Journal of the American Geriatrics Society* 21 (6) 1973: 253–55.

Village Voice. "Food in Thought." May 31, 1976: 19.

Villas, Tennyson. Letter to Jerome Agel, March 1, 1976.

W. "The Delights of Fasting." Nov. 14–21, 1975: 24–25.

Walsh, C. H., et al. "Effect of Different Periods of Fasting on Oral Glucose Tolerance." *British Medical Journal* 2 (5868) 1973: 691–93.

Walter, R. D., et al. "The Effect of Adrenergic Blockade on the Glucagon Responses to Starvation and Hypoglycemia in Man." *Journal of Clinical Investigation* 54 (5) 1974: 1214–20.

Ward, Jack T. Letter to Jerome Agel, March 1, 1976.

Washington Post, The. "The Price of Meat." June 21, 1975: A 12.

Waters, Enoc P. "Plentiful Protein from the Sea." *FDA Consumer,* Nov. 1973.

Weber, Melva. "Weight-Loss Fast." *Vogue,* Jan. 1976: 107+.

Weinberg, Alfred F. Letter to Jerome Agel (undated).

Wesselhoeft, Conrad. "The Lewis and Clark Expedition Into Natural Foods." *Prevention,* April 1976: 126–31.

Wetzel, Betty. Letters to Jerome Agel from Oxfam-America, April 27 and May 1, 1976.

White, Philip L. "At Last, the Ultimate Diet: Total Fasting (Total Foolishness)." *American Medical News,* Jan. 19, 1976: 4.

Wigmore, Ann. Letters to Jerome Agel, Jan. 26 and March 5, 1976.

Wilhelmi, H. Ph. Letter to Jerome Agel, April 15, 1976.

Willard, Jo. Letters to Jerome Agel, March 23 and April 15, 1976.

Williams, Tennessee. *Memoirs.* New York: Doubleday, 1975.

Winakor, Bess. "The Most Restrictive Diet: Just Don't Eat—Anything." *Chicago Sun-Times,* Aug. 19, 1975: 33.

Women's Wear Daily. "At Shrubland Hall." March 14, 1975: 13.

———. "Faster, Faster." Feb. 13, 1976.

Wren, Christopher S. "Soviet Jew, Denied Exit, Continues Fast." *The New York Times,* April 21, 1975.

Yogananda, Paramahansa. "The Physical and Spiritual Rewards of Fasting." Self-Realization Fellowship, Los Angeles, Calif.

Youmans, John B. "Hunger and Malnutrition." Letter to the Editor, *Journal of the American Medical Association* 214 (6) 1970: 1123.

Young, V. R., et al. "Potential Use of 3-Methylhistidine Excretion as an Index of Progressive Reduction in Muscle Protein Catabolism during Starvation." *Metabolism: Clinical and Experimental* 22 (11) 1973: 1429–36.

———. "Protein Requirements of Man: Comparative Nitrogen Balance Response within the Submaintenance-to-maintenance Range of Intakes of Wheat and Beef Proteins." *Journal of Nutrition* 105 (5) 1975: 534–42.

In addition, there were innumerable interviews with and correspondence from patients of Dr. Cott.

ABOUT THE AUTHORS

ALLAN COTT, M.D., author of *Fasting: The Ultimate Diet*, a psychiatrist in private practice in New York City and on the attending staff, Gracie Square Hospital, where he fasted patients. A Life Fellow of the American Psychiatric Association, Founding Fellow and President of the Academy of Orthomolecular Psychiatry, Consultant to the Allan Cott School for children with severe disorders of behavior, communication, and learning, and Consultant to the Spear Educational Center for severely disturbed children. Author of many articles on the treatment of mental illness in adults and on the treatment of seriously disturbed children and learning disabled children with the use of vitamins, minerals and dietary control. With Jerome Agel and Eugene Boe, he authored *Dr. Cott's Help for Your Learning Disabled Child*.

JEROME AGEL, co-author of *Fasting: The Ultimate Diet*, has been involved in fifty major books as author, co-author, and/ or producer. They include *22 Fires* (a novel); *The Cosmic Connection* and *Other Worlds* (with Carl Sagan); *Herman Kahnsciousness; The Making of Kubrick's 2001; The Medium is the Massage* (with Marshall McLuhan); *It's About Time & It's About Time* (with Alan Lakein); *Understanding Understanding* (with Humphry Osmond); and *I Seem to Be a Verb* (with Buckminster Fuller). Since first publication of this book, in 1972, he has written *Why in the World* (with George J. Demko), *Pearls of Wisdom, Amending America* (with Richard B. Bernstein), *Cleopatra's Nose*, and *Between Columbus and the Pilgrims: The Americas 1492–1620*.

EUGENE BOE, co-author of *Fasting: The Ultimate Diet*, co-authored or contributed to many books, including *The Immigrant Experience, Hart's Guide to New York City*, and *Cooking Creatively with Natural Foods*. He is the co-author with Jerome Agel of the non-fiction novels *22 Fires* and *Deliverance in Shanghai*.

HUMIRA
OTEZLA
ENBREL